rvw 7/17

COMPLETE M

D1586591

IN PSYCHIA

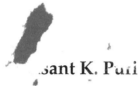

...sant K. Puri

C..sultant & Senior Lecturer,
Imp..ial College School of Medicine,
Hammersmith Hospital,
London, UK

Anne D. Hall

Consultant Psychiatrist,
South Kensington and Chelsea Mental Health Centre,
Chelsea & Westminster Hospital,
London, UK

ARNOLD

A member of the Hodder Headline Group
LONDON • SYDNEY • AUCKLAND
Co-published in the USA by Oxford University Press Inc., New York

First published in Great Britain in 1999 by
Arnold, a division of Hodder Headline PLC,
338 Euston Road, London NW1 3BH
http://www.arnoldpublishers.com

Co-published in the United States of America by
Oxford University Press Inc.,
198 Madison Avenue, New York, NY 10016

British Library Cataloguing in Publication Data
A catalogue entry for this book is available from the British Library

Library of Congress Cataloging-in-Publication Data
A catalog record for this book is available from the Library of Congress

ISBN 0 340 74035 3

1 2 3 4 5 95 96 97 98 99

Publisher: Georgina Bentliff
Production Editor: James Rabson
Production Controller: Sarah Kett
Cover designer: Terry Griffiths

Typeset in 10/12 pt Helvetica by Prepress Projects, Perth, Scotland
Printed and bound in the United Kingdom by J.W. Arrowsmith Ltd, Bristol

What do you think about this book? Or any other
Arnold title? Please send your comments to
feedback.arnold@hodder.co.uk

Contents

PREFACE

This book of multiple-choice questions (MCQs) is a companion to our *Revision Notes in Psychiatry* [1] with the individual chapters of the two books matching. The MCQs follow the format currently used by the Royal College of Psychiatrists for the MRCPsych examinations. Each question consists of a stem or introductory statement followed by five items, labelled A to E, each of which may be true or false. One mark is obtained for each item answered correctly, and one mark deducted for each item answered incorrectly.

We have attempted to cover the whole of psychiatry, including the sciences basic to psychiatry, and for each question we have given explanations of the answers, in as much detail as we consider appropriate, together with references, usually to the relevant part of *Revision Notes in Psychiatry*. It is recommended that all the questions in a given chapter be attempted before checking the answers to that chapter, and that the material underlying any questions answered incorrectly be revised carefully if the reasons for the errors are not immediately understood. In this way we hope that working through the chapters of this book will prove useful both as an aid to consolidating understanding and knowledge during the study process, and as a revision in the weeks leading to examinations. Those taking examinations other than in postgraduate psychiatry may also find this book of use through the selective choice of chapters.

BKP
ADH

[1] Puri, B.K. and Hall, A.D. (1998) *Revision Notes in Psychiatry*. London: Arnold.

REFERENCES

Atkinson, R.L., Atkinson, R.C. and Hilgard, E.R. (1983) *Introduction to Psychology,* 8th edn. San Diego: Harcourt Brace Jovanovich.

Johnson, M.H. and Everitt, B.J. (1995) *Essential Reproduction,* 4th edn. Oxford: Blackwell Science.

Lishman, W.A. (1998) *Organic Psychiatry: the Psychological Consequences of Cerebral Disorder,* 3rd edn. Oxford: Blackwell Science.

Puri, B.K. and Tyrer, P.J. (1992) *Sciences Basic to Psychiatry,* 1st edn. Edinburgh: Churchill Livingstone.

Puri, B.K. and Hall, A.D. (1998) *Revision Notes in Psychiatry.* London: Arnold.

Puri, B.K. and Tyrer, P.J. (1998) *Sciences Basic to Psychiatry,* 2nd edn. Edinburgh: Churchill Livingstone.

Puri, B.K., Laking, P.J. and Treasaden, I.H. (1996) *Textbook of Psychiatry.* London: Churchill Livingstone.

Tantam, D. and Birchwood, M. (eds) (1994) *Seminars in Psychology and the Social Sciences.* London: Gaskell.

PART ONE

Questions

1 Basic Psychology

Questions

1.1 Cognitive dissonance:

   A is a cause of internal discomfort
   B is associated with decreased arousal
   C was first described by McClelland
   D is the term used to describe the situation when attitude and behaviour are inconsistent
   E can lead to a change in behaviour

1.2 Operant conditioning is:

   A useful in the management of children with learning difficulties
   B a form of classical conditioning
   C based on techniques derived from hypnosis
   D sometimes achieved by using punishment as a form of negative reinforcement
   E achieved with a higher response rate when built up under continuous reinforcement rather than partial reinforcement with a fixed interval schedule

1.3 Behaviour therapy may use the following concepts:

   A habituation
   B imprinting
   C reciprocal inhibition
   D shaping
   E chaining

1.4 Optimal conditions for vicarious learning include:

   A escape conditioning
   B reinforcement
   C maximum likelihood estimation
   D drug-induced behavioural change
   E perceived similarity

1.5 Perceptual phenomena described in Gestalt psychology include:

   A the law of effect
   B the law of simplicity
   C the law of proximity
   D figure ground differentiation
   E Fechner's law

1.6   Depth perception:

   A   is usually present at birth
   B   involves object interposition
   C   may be demonstrated using the visual cliff
   D   may be abnormal in schizophrenia
   E   may be abnormal in derealization

1.7   The following aspects of visual perception are believed to be innate:

   A   figure ground discrimination
   B   haptic memory
   C   fixating
   D   size constancy
   E   shape discrimination

1.8   Processes that are primarily related to attention rather than to memory include:

   A   the recency effect
   B   decay
   C   the Stroop effect
   D   dual-task interference
   E   chunking

1.9   Types of memory that are primarily part of long-term memory include:

   A   primary memory
   B   echoic memory
   C   sensory memory
   D   episodic memory
   E   working memory

1.10   Secondary drives:

   A   may result from generalization
   B   may result from conditioning
   C   include thirst
   D   include anxiety
   E   refer to a concept developed primarily by Hull

1.11   Theories of intrinsic motivation include:

   A optimal arousal
   B drive reduction
   C need for achievement
   D cognitive dissonance
   E attitude-discrepant behaviour

1.12   The following have put forward theories relating to the experience of emotion:

   A James
   B Lange
   C Cannon
   D Bard
   E Schachter

1.13   Primary emotions:

   A include love
   B include disgust
   C include submission
   D in combinations of two, can give rise to secondary emotions
   E were classified by Plutchik

1.14   The following coping mechanisms are correctly paired with the corresponding unconscious defence mechanisms to which they relate:

   A empathy–repression
   B concentration only on the current task– denial
   C logical analysis–rationalization
   D objectivity–reaction formation
   E playfulness–regression

2 SOCIAL PSYCHOLOGY

Questions

2.1 Attitudes:

   A may be measured using a Likert scale
   B are based on beliefs
   C have affective components
   D are mutually consistent
   E are based on a tendency to behave in an observable way

2.2 The likelihood that communications will be persuasive for a recipient of high intelligence is increased in the following cases:

   A the message is repeated
   B the message is explicit rather than implicit
   C the communicator is an opinion leader
   D interactive personal discussion rather than mass media communication takes place
   E one-sided communication rather than two-sided presentations takes place

2.3 Theories of interpersonal attraction include:

   A balance theory
   B equity theory
   C attribution theory
   D reinforcement theory
   E proxemics

2.4 Types of social power include:

   A referent
   B coercive
   C normative
   D authority
   E expert

2.5 The following conditions are likely to reduce prejudice:

   A situational attribution
   B cooperative effort
   C maintaining a distance
   D equal status
   E exposure to non-stereotypic individuals

3 NEUROPSYCHOLOGY

Questions

3.1 Explicit memory:

A is a type of short-term memory
B is recalled automatically without effort
C is amenable to verbal reporting
D includes episodic memory
E requires the medial temporal lobes to be intact

3.2 The following statements concerning implicit memory are true:

A it is learnt relatively slowly
B learning usually requires repetition
C it primarily comprises factual knowledge
D it requires the cerebellum to be intact
E it is involved in operant learning

3.3 The following statements concerning language are true:

A in most left-handers the right cerebral hemisphere is dominant
B cerebral dominance is fixed at birth
C an inability to read is a characteristic feature of lesions of the angular gyrus
D an inability to write is a characteristic feature of lesions of the angular gyrus
E the auditory association cortex is found mainly in the frontal lobe of the dominant hemisphere

3.4 Damage confined to Wernicke's area is characteristically associated with:

A speech that is abnormal in intonation
B speech that is abnormal in rhythm
C expressive dysphasia
D loss of the ability to understand the written word
E paraphasias

3.5 Damage confined to the arcuate fasciculus is characteristically associated with:

A a conduction dysphasia
B disruption of the ability to comprehend spoken language
C intact verbal fluency
D an inability to repeat what is said
E aggressive behaviour

3.6   Functions solely of the occipital lobes in visual perception include the determination
      of the following aspects of objects:

      A   shape
      B   colour
      C   complete percepts
      D   spatial orientation
      E   meaning

3.7   The following brain regions and agnosias characteristically associated with lesions
      of those regions are correctly paired:

      A   occipital lobes–apperceptive visual agnosia
      B   non-dominant parietal lobe–anosognosia
      C   dominant temporal lobe–associative agnosia
      D   Broca's area–expressive dysphasia
      E   lingual gyri–achromatopsia

3.8   The following statements concerning apraxias are correct:

      A   apraxia may result from sensory loss
      B   apraxia may result from paresis
      C   in ideational apraxia there is an inability to carry out a coordinated sequence of
          actions
      D   in ideomotor apraxia there is an inability to carry out progressively difficult tasks
      E   in constructional apraxia there is an inability to construct a figure

3.9   The following statements concerning agnosias are correct:

      A   in simultanagnosia there is an inability to name, recognize or point on command
          to parts of the body
      B   in agnosia for colours, colour sense is absent
      C   the presence of prosopagnosia may be inferred from the mirror sign
      D   the presence of astereognosia is tested using a locomotor map-reading task in
          which the patient is asked to trace out a given route by foot
      E   agraphaesthesia is tested by asking the patient to identify, with closed eyes,
          numbers or letters traced on their palm

3.10 Gerstmann's syndrome:

      A   characteristically results from non-dominant parietal lobe lesions
      B   includes right–left disorientation
      C   includes aphasia
      D   includes finger agnosia
      E   includes dyscalculia

3.11   Functions more likely to be associated with the prefrontal cortex than the orbital
       cortex include:

       A   social behaviour
       B   memory
       C   verbal regulation
       D   problem-solving
       E   personality

3.12   Frontal lobe lesions may give rise to:

       A   pallilalia
       B   sensory fits
       C   urinary incontinence
       D   personality change
       E   ipsilateral optic atrophy

4 PSYCHOLOGICAL ASSESSMENT

Questions

4.1 The following definitions of sources of error in psychological assessment by interview are correct:

A scaling – conversion of raw data into types of scores more readily understood
B Hawthorne effect – the subject avoids giving too much self-related information
C response set – the choice of responses that the subject believes the interviewer desires
D extreme responding – the tendency always to agree or to disagree with the questions asked
E halo effect – the tendency always to avoid extreme responses

4.2 The following statements concerning measurement in psychological assessment are correct:

A naturalistic observations are used in the functional analysis of problem behaviours
B defensiveness is a potential source of error
C norm-referencing and criterion-referencing may be used
D social desirability may be reduced by using the forced-choice technique
E social desirability may be reduced by including a lie scale

4.3 Tests of intelligence in adults include:

A WPPSI
B WISC-R
C CHAID
D WAIS
E the Stanford–Binet test

4.4 The following statements concerning subtests of the WAIS-R are correct:

A there are five verbal subtests
B there are five performance subtests
C vocabulary is a subtest
D digit span is a subtest
E digit symbol is a subtest

4.5   Projective tests of personality include:

A   California Psychological Inventory
B   Thematic Apperception Test
C   Rorschach Inkblot Test
D   Minnesota Multiphasic Personality Inventory
E   Sentence Completion Test

5 HUMAN DEVELOPMENT

Questions

5.1 Individuals who have devised stage theories of human development include:

A Kohlberg
B Spearman
C Piaget
D Sigmund Freud
E Erikson

5.2 The following important aspects of attachment during early development are correctly paired with individuals with whom they are associated:

A contact comfort–Harlow
B imprinting–Lorenz
C avoidant attachment–Tanner
D transitional object–Anna Freud
E attachment theory–Bowlby

5.3 Attachment:

A usually takes place from mother to infant
B is more commonly evident in its polytropic rather than its monotropic form
C may be considered to result from the mother acting as a conditioned reinforcer
D takes an average of 10 months to become fully established
E is reinforced by crying

5.4 Characteristic features of acute separation reactions in infants who have started to form attachments include:

A despair
B grief
C alarm
D detachment
E protest

5.5 Recognized effects of maternal deprivation include:

A poor growth
B chronic fatigue syndrome
C developmental language delay
D increased empathy with others
E enuresis

5.6 The following phenomena are features associated with dysfunctional families:

A social desirability
B triangulation
C enmeshment
D disengagement
E the creation of myths

5.7 Recognized sequelae of child sexual abuse include:

A increased control of sexual impulses
B strengthened gender identity
C dissociation
D eating disorders
E reduced incidence of homosexuality

5.8 Recognized sequelae of childhood physical abuse include:

A depression
B schizophrenia
C personality disorder
D neurological impairment
E delayed language development

5.9 The following features of cognitive development are characteristically associated with the sensorimotor stage:

A tertiary circular reactions
B reversibility
C egocentrism
D conservation of number
E object permanence

5.10 The preoperational stage of cognitive development:

A occurs from age 7 to around 12–14 years
B is one in which thought processes include authoritarian morality
C is one of Kohlberg's stages of development
D is one in which thought processes include creationism
E is characterized by the inability to test hypotheses systematically

5.11   By the age of 8 months, a normally developing infant:

        A   typically has a vocabulary of four or five words
        B   exhibits tertiary circular reactions
        C   exhibits authority orientation
        D   shows a fear of heights
        E   is in the anal phase of psychosexual development

5.12   The following are associated with slower speech development during childhood:

        A   being female
        B   being one of twins
        C   prolonged second-stage labour
        D   larger family size
        E   a bilingual home

5.13   In Kohlberg's stage theory of moral development, conventional morality:

        A   is level I
        B   includes reward orientation
        C   includes good-boy/good-girl orientation
        D   has three stages
        E   is typically seen in children aged up to about 6 or 7 years

5.14   Fear of the following typically begins at around 3 years of age:

        A   strangers
        B   monsters
        C   ridicule
        D   failure
        E   the dark

5.15   The following have a masculinizing effect during ontogeny:

        A   SRY
        B   over-ripeness of the ovum at fertilization
        C   21-hydroxylase deficiency
        D   absence of fetal androgen
        E   a reduced number of primordial germ cells

5.16   Pubic hair growth during puberty:

        A   follows adrenarche
        B   is usually the first sign of the onset of puberty in girls
        C   is usually the first sign of the onset of puberty in boys
        D   can be recorded using a standardized system devised by Tanner
        E   is usually normal in Turner's syndrome

5.17 The following statements concerning normal sexual development are true:

A gender identity refers to the type of behaviour that an individual engages in that identifies him or her as being male or female
B gender identity is usually established by the age of 1.5 to 2 years
C once established, gender identity usually remains unchanged
D gender typing is the process by which individuals acquire a sense of gender and gender-related cultural traits appropriate to the society and age into which they are born
E parents play a major role in sex typing

5.18 Findings by Offer and Offer from their study of American men who were adolescents during the 1960s showed that these adolescents:

A often abused heroin
B generally held basic values that differed significantly from those of their parents
C came mainly from intact families
D usually engaged in major delinquent behaviour
E usually went on to college

5.19 Adolescent developmental routes identified by Offer and Offer include:

A retarded growth
B continuous growth
C ego-resilient growth
D surgent growth
E tumultuous growth

5.20 Groups of female adolescents identified by Block and Haan using factor analysis include:

A cognitive type
B belated adjusters
C hyperfeminine repressors
D dominant narcissists
E lonely independents

5.21 The following symptoms are more likely to indicate a normal grief reaction than a depressive disorder:

A hallucinations of the deceased
B a morbid preoccupation with worthlessness
C numbness
D the feeling that one should have died with the deceased person
E marked psychoactive retardation

5.22   The following are more likely to indicate a morbid grief reaction rather than normal
        grief:

        A   irritability
        B   early morning wakening
        C   identification phenomena
        D   delay of reaction
        E   denial of anger

6 PRINCIPLES OF EVALUATION AND PSYCHOMETRICS

Questions

6.1 In a psychometric study of working adults, a variable is created that corresponds to the social class of these individuals. This variable:

   A   is qualitative
   B   is measured on an interval scale
   C   is discrete
   D   has at least five values
   E   follows a normal distribution

6.2 Variables that can be measured using a ratio scale include:

   A   the number of previous inpatient psychiatric admissions
   B   body temperature (in °C)
   C   height (in m)
   D   body mass (in kg)
   E   hair colour

6.3 Types of sampling methods that can be used in psychiatric research include:

   A   nominal
   B   periodic
   C   stratified
   D   systematic
   E   simple

6.4 The following probability distributions are continuous:

   A   chi-squared
   B   Bernoulli
   C   binomial
   D   normal
   E F

6.5 If the IQ of a population of individuals follows a normal distribution with mean 100 and standard deviation 15, then the following are true:

   A   the median is 100
   B   the variance is 15
   C   the area under the probability density function curve is greater than 10
   D   the mode is 1
   E   over two-thirds of the population have an IQ in the range 85–115 (inclusive)

6.6   The following are properties of the normal distribution probability density function curve:

    A   it is bimodal
    B   the median is equal to the mode
    C   the area between the mean and two standard deviations greater than the mean encloses approximately 95% of the total area under the curve
    D   the two-tailed 5% points are given by $\mu \pm 1.96\sigma$
    E   the standard normal distribution has approximately the same probability density function curve as the *t* distribution with over 30 degrees of freedom

6.7   The ages (in years) of a sample of four children with AD/HD are 4, 8, 8 and 10. The following statements are correct:

    A   the mean is 7.5 years
    B   the median is 7.5 years
    C   the mode is 8 years
    D   the variance is 8.4 years
    E   the range is 6 years

6.8   Outliers:

    A   may be detected by graphical methods
    B   are likely to have a greater effect on the median than on the mean, particularly when the total number of values is small
    C   may affect the range to a lesser extent than they affect the standard deviation
    D   may exert an extreme effect on the correlation coefficient
    E   may exert an extreme effect on the results of linear regression

6.9   The following statements concerning boxplots, the longer sides of which are placed vertically, are correct:

    A   they can be used to compare two or more sets of continuous observations diagrammatically
    B   the length of the box represents the range
    C   the upper boundary of the box represents the mean plus one standard deviation
    D   the horizontal line inside the box represents the mean
    E   they are also known as stem-and-leaf plots

6.10   The following are examples of descriptive statistics:

    A   diagrammatic representations of data
    B   graphical representations of data
    C   *P*-values
    D   95% confidence intervals
    E   data expressed in the form of a table

6.11   A hypothesis test is carried out in which the unknown parameter θ is hypothesized under the null hypothesis to take the value θ_0. Composite hypotheses include:

  A $\theta = \theta_0$
  B $\theta = \theta_1$, where $\theta_1 \neq \theta_0$
  C $\theta \neq \theta_0$
  D $\theta > \theta_0$
  E $\theta < \theta_0$

6.12   A statistical test is carried out to determine whether the mean haemoglobin level of a group of male outpatients with schizophrenia (12.2 g dl^{-1}) differs from that of a comparison group of an equal number of age-matched male control subjects (14.0 g dl^{-1}). The two-sided 95% confidence interval for this difference is calculated to be -2.1 to 2.3 g dl^{-1}. This implies that:

  A $P < 0.05$
  B   the probability of a type I error is 0.05
  C   there is a 95% chance that the difference lies between -2.1 and 2.3 g dl^{-1}
  D   there is no evidence to suggest that the haemoglobin levels of the two groups differ significantly
  E   the one-sided 95% confidence interval for the difference is 0 to approximately 2.3 g dl^{-1}

6.13   Referring to the previous question (6.12), the following statistical tests could be used to calculate whether the haemoglobin levels differ significantly between the two groups (which are matched in terms of age, sex and number):

  A   paired *t*-test
  B   chi-squared test
  C   ANOVA
  D   Mann–Whitney *U*-test
  E   Levene's test

6.14   A chi-squared test on a 3×3 contingency table:

  A   is a parametric test
  B   can use Yates' continuity correction
  C   can be replaced by Fisher's exact probability test
  D   has one degree of freedom
  E   is only valid if each expected value is at least 5

6.15   The following statements concerning clinical trials carried out by the pharmaceutical industry are correct:

    A the gold standard for such trials is the randomized double-blind controlled trial
    B clinical trials include post-marketing surveillance
    C initial pharmacological investigations are carried out in phase II trials
    D a full-scale treatment evaluation is carried out in phase IV trials
    E toxicity studies are carried out in phase I trials

6.16   Latent traits:

    A are usually directly observable
    B may be identified using factor analysis
    C may be used to make predictions
    D include intelligence
    E include attitude

6.17   Reliability in psychiatric measurement:

    A describes whether a test or measuring instrument measures what it purports to measure
    B can be expressed as the ratio of the variance of the true scores to the variance of the observed scores
    C ranges from −1 to 1 (inclusive)
    D includes an alternative forms type
    E includes a split-half type

6.18   Statistical tests of reliability include:

    A percentage agreement
    B product-moment correlation coefficient
    C kappa statistic
    D intraclass correlation coefficient
    E Cronbach's α

6.19   The following are types of validity:

    A content
    B predictive
    C face
    D inter-rater
    E construct

6.20   The following statements concerning measurement in psychiatry are correct:

A a type II error is the probability that the null hypothesis is rejected when it is indeed false

B a type I error is the power of a test

C a type I error is denoted by α

D the specificity of a test is the proportion of positive results or cases correctly identified

E the predictive value of a negative result from a research measure is the proportion of the negative results that is true negative

6.21   Types of bias include:

A recall

B convergent

C selection

D concurrent

E information

6.22   The following statements concerning statistical tests are true:

A meta-analysis is an attempt to express a set of multivariate data as a linear function of unobserved, underlying dimensions, or factors together with error terms

B publication bias may be an important confounding factor in a meta-analysis

C a survival curve may be drawn in a stepwise fashion

D the hazard function measures the likelihood of an individual experiencing a given event as a function of time

E a logistic regression model predicts the probability of a continuous dependent variable on the basis of a set of continuous independent variables

7 SOCIAL SCIENCES

Questions

7.1   The following statements concerning social class are true:

   A   the type of residence lived in is a determinant of social class
   B   leisure activities are a determinant of social class
   C   semi-skilled occupations are classified as social class III in Britain (Office of Population Censuses and Surveys)
   D   the unemployed are classified as social class V in Britain (Office of Population Censuses and Surveys)
   E   members of the same household are assigned to the social class of the head of the household in Britain (Office of Population Censuses and Surveys)

7.2   The following disorders are more likely to be diagnosed in upper social classes than in lower ones:

   A   alcohol dependence
   B   heroin dependence
   C   personality disorder
   D   anorexia nervosa in women
   E   bulimia nervosa in women

7.3   The following disorders are more likely to be diagnosed in lower social classes than in upper ones:

   A   schizophrenia
   B   organic psychosis
   C   bipolar mood disorder
   D   depressive episodes in women
   E   parasuicide

7.4   Filters to psychiatric care:

   A   depend in part on service provision
   B   depend in part on the patient's age
   C   depend in part on the severity of the disorder
   D   include the decision by the patient to consult their general practitioner
   E   include recognition of the disorder by the general practitioner

7.5 The social role of doctors:

    A was first described by Mechanic
    B includes obligations
    C includes legitimizing illness
    D includes defining illness
    E includes imposing an illness diagnosis if necessary

7.6 Scales of the Camberwell Family Interview that are associated with high expressed emotion include:

    A positive remarks
    B double-bind
    C critical comments
    D marital schism
    E emotional overinvolvement

7.7 The following factors relating to family life are correctly paired with the persons who first described them in relation to major mental illness:

    A schizophrenogenic mother–Dare
    B double-bind–Bateson
    C marital skew–Vaughn and Leff
    D abnormal family communication–Wynne *et al.*
    E expressed emotion–Gruzelier

7.8 The following statements regarding life events are correct:

    A marital separation is a life event that has a relatively high (greater than 50) life-change value
    B the Life Events and Difficulties Schedule was devised by Holmes and Rahe
    C there is strong evidence that threatening life events are more common before the first onset of mania
    D there Is strong evidence that threatening life events are more common before self-poisoning attempts
    E the death of one's spouse has a lower life-change value than does a gaol term

7.9 Vulnerability factors identified by Brown and Harris that make a woman more susceptible to suffer from depression following life events include:

    A having a mother who was overtly hostile to her as a child
    B the loss of her mother before the age of 11 years
    C not working outside the home
    D being aloof from her child(ren)
    E having one or more child(ren) under the age of 13 years at home

7.10   The following statements concerning total institutions are correct:

   A   older large psychiatric hospitals are examples of total institutions
   B   western democratic political parties are examples of total institutions
   C   a total institution is defined as an established and sanctioned form of relationship between social beings
   D   the total institution is a concept introduced by Goffman
   E   the mortification process is the process whereby an individual becomes an inhabitant of a total institution

7.11   Reactions that occur to the mortification process include:

   A   withdrawal
   B   colonization
   C   open rebellion
   D   conversion
   E   institutionalization

8 Descriptive Psychopathology

Questions

8.1 The following movement disorders may occur in patients with schizophrenia:

A ambitendency
B dysprosody
C schizophasia
D negativism
E echopraxia

8.2 The following disorders appear to be goal directed:

A thought blocking
B stereotypies
C circumstantiality
D tics
E mannerisms

8.3 Types of perseveration of speech include:

A logorrhoea
B drivelling
C vorbeigehen
D palilalia
E logoclonia

8.4 Connections between thoughts in flight of ideas may be based on:

A assonance
B chance relationships
C distracting stimuli
D clang associations
E alliteration

8.5 Features of formal thought disorder described by Schneider include:

A derealization
B depersonalization
C fusion
D omission
E substitution

8.6   Examples of delusions include:

   A   Othello syndrome
   B   l'illusion de sosies
   C   somatic passivity
   D   ideas of reference
   E   erotomania

8.7   The following are sensory deceptions rather than sensory distortions:

   A   hyperacusis
   B   xanthopsia
   C   autoscopy
   D   trailing phenomenon
   E   micropsia

8.8   The following are receptive aphasias:

   A   syntactical aphasia
   B   agnosic alexia
   C   pure word deafness
   D   visual asymbolia
   E   nominal aphasia

9 PSYCHOANALYTIC THEORIES

Questions

9.1 In Freud's topographical model of the mind, the preconscious:

  A uses primary process thinking
  B is timeless
  C is word oriented
  D is non-linear
  E is within awareness

9.2 The unconscious, in Freud's topographical model of the mind, is:

  A declarative
  B motivated by the reality principle
  C symbolic
  D timeless
  E image oriented

9.3 Attributes of primary process thinking as described by Freud include:

  A delayed gratification
  B symbolization
  C condensation
  D secondary elaboration
  E displacement

9.4 In Freudian psychoanalytic theory, components of the latent dream include:

  A nocturnal stimuli
  B secondary revision
  C the day residue
  D dream work
  E unconscious wishes

9.5 Instinctual drives identified by Freud include:

  A transference
  B eros
  C id
  D thanatos
  E libido

9.6   According to Sigmund Freud, the following statements concerning the phallic phase of psychosexual development are correct:

A   it typically occurs from 15 – 18 months to 30 – 36 months of age
B   erotogenic pleasure is derived primarily from sucking
C   boys pass through the Oedipal complex during this phase
D   girls develop penis envy during this phase
E   girls pass through the Electra complex during this phase

9.7   Types of archetype identified in Jungian theory include the:

A   animus
B   inferiority complex
C   shadow
D   self
E   persona

9.8   The following concepts are associated with Jungian theory rather than Freudian theory:

A   teleology
B   countertransference
C   superego
D   synchronicity
E   pleasure principle

9.9   The development of the paranoid–schizoid position in Kleinian theory is particularly associated with the following defence mechanisms:

A   introjection
B   intellectualization
C   splitting
D   projective identification
E   denial

9.10   Psychoanalytic concepts associated with Melanie Klein include:

A   transitional object
B   depressive position
C   oral sadism
D   oral envy
E   castration anxiety

9.11   Concepts associated with Winnicott include:

   A objective countertransference
   B good-enough mother
   C capacity to be alone
   D squiggle game
   E holding environment

10 NEUROANATOMY

Questions

10.1 The following structures are correctly paired with the neural tube vesicles from which they derive during embryological development:

  A cerebellum–rhombencephalon
  B pineal gland–mesencephalon
  C pons–myelencephalon
  D rhinencephalon–telencephalon
  E superior colliculi–diencephalon

10.2 The following statements concerning neurones are true:

  A in bipolar neurones the perikaryon has just one neurite
  B multipolar neurones each have one axon and more than one dendrite
  C Schwann cells are predominantly found in the peripheral nervous system rather than the central nervous system
  D Golgi type II neurones have relatively long axons
  E amacrine neurones have short axons that terminate near the parent cell

10.3 The following are central nervous system neuroglia:

  A tanycytes
  B satellite cells
  C protoplasmic astrocytes
  D microglia
  E oligodendrocytes

10.4 The following statements concerning the frontal operculum are correct:

  A it contains the orbital cortex
  B it contains the supplementary motor area
  C it contains the anterior cingulate cortex
  D it contains areas 44 and 45
  E lesions in the non-dominant side are associated with dysprosody

10.5 Lesions of the dorsolateral prefrontal cortex are associated with:

  A impaired verbal fluency
  B expressive aphasia
  C disturbances in motor programming
  D poor abstraction
  E poor organization

10.6   The mesial temporal region contains the:

    A   angular gyrus
    B   amygdala
    C   hippocampus
    D   entorhinal cortex
    E   supramarginal gyrus

10.7   Balint's syndrome:

    A   includes simultanagnosia
    B   includes prosopagnosia
    C   includes psychic gaze paralysis
    D   includes receptive aphasia
    E   follows temporoparietal junction lesions on the dominant side

10.8   Components of the basal ganglia include the:

    A   globus pallidus
    B   amygdala
    C   parahippocampal gyrus
    D   claustrum
    E   corpus striatum

10.9   Efferents from the globus pallidus pass directly to the:

    A   substantia nigra
    B   ventroanterior nucleus of the thalamus
    C   reticular formation
    D   hypothalamus
    E   subthalamus

10.10   Alexander's frontal–subcortical circuits include the following circuits:

    A   motor
    B   sensory
    C   oculomotor
    D   limbic
    E   medial orbitofrontal

10.11   Cortical areas of the limbic lobe include the:

    A   cingulate gyrus
    B   amygdala
    C   hippocampus gyrus
    D   fornix
    E   subcallosal gyrus

10.12   The following cortical areas are part of the limbic system:

        A   orbital cortex
        B   prepiriform cortex
        C   subcallosal gyrus
        D   Broca's area
        E   subiculum

10.13   The following subcortical nuclear groups are part of the limbic system:

        A   anterior thalamic nucleus
        B   pretectal nucleus
        C   main oculomotor nucleus
        D   mammillary body
        E   dendate nucleus

10.14   Connecting pathways of the limbic system include the:

        A   cingulum
        B   stria terminalis
        C   fornix
        D   arcuate bundle
        E   dorsal longitudinal fasciculus

10.15   Major divisions of the corpus callosum include the:

        A   rostrum
        B   septum
        C   indusium
        D   granum
        E   body

10.16   Components of the Papez circuit include the:

        A   dorsomedial nucleus of the thalamus
        B   cingulate gyrus
        C   fornix
        D   habenular nucleus
        E   hypothalamus

10.17   The oculomotor nerve:

        A   carries parasympathetic fibres
        B   supplies the superior oblique muscle
        C   runs close to the apex of the petrous temporal bone
        D   is the sixth cranial nerve
        E   if divided results in ptosis

10.18 The superior raphe nuclei:

    A give rise to ascending fibres that project to the forebrain
    B include the suprachiasmatic nucleus
    C include the caudal linear nucleus
    D include the supralemniscal nucleus
    E form the main noradrenergic nuclei in the central nervous system

11 NEUROPATHOLOGY

Questions

11.1 The following macroscopic neuropathological changes are more likely to be seen in the brain in Alzheimer's disease than in Pick's disease:

   A global atrophy
   B ventricular enlargement
   C depigmentation of the substantia nigra
   D senile plaques
   E knife-blade gyri

11.2 The following are characteristically seen in the hippocampus in Alzheimer's disease:

   A neurofibrillary tangles
   B neuritic plaques
   C Hirano bodies
   D Lewy bodies
   E granulovacuolar degeneration

11.3 Pick's bodies:

   A contain dense core vesicles
   B have an amyloid core
   C contain straight neurofilaments
   D contain paired helical filaments
   E are characteristically found in the locus coeruleus in Pick's disease

11.4 Lewy bodies:

   A contain dense core vesicles
   B contain neurofibrillary tangles
   C contain tau protein
   D contain ubiquitin
   E are characteristically found in Parkinson's disease

11.5 Neuropathological changes characteristically seen in those surviving the longest with Creutzfeldt–Jakob disease include:

A cerebral atrophy
B ventricular enlargement
C perforation of the septum pellucidum
D thinning of the corpus callosum
E status spongiosus

11.6 Neurilemmomas:

A are derived from blood vessels
B are also known as Schwannomas
C include ependymomas
D include acoustic neuromas
E have a higher incidence than cerebral metastases

11.7 Gross neuropathological changes characteristically found in the brains of patients with schizophrenia compared with normal controls include:

A increased brain length
B decreased white matter volume
C decreased grey matter volume
D decreased brain mass
E ventricular enlargement

11.8 Temporal lobe changes characteristically found in schizophrenia include:

A reduced hippocampal surface area
B decreased grey matter in the anterior hippocampus
C pyramidal cell disorientation in the hippocampus
D increased neuronal size in the entorhinal cortex
E significant gliosis

11.9 The following neuropathological changes are correctly paired with the disorders in which they characteristically occur:

A loss of dopaminergic neurones in the substantia nigra–Huntington's disease
B atrophy of the neostriatum–tardive dyskinesia
C depigmentation of the locus coeruleus–idiopathic Parkinson's disease
D increased Purkinje cell count in the cerebellum–autism
E knife-blade gyri–Pick's disease

12 NEUROIMAGING TECHNIQUES

Questions

12.1   Magnetic resonance scanners can be used to obtain the following information about the brain:

   A   high-resolution structural images
   B   neuronal membrane phospholipid metabolism
   C   the concentration of fluorine-containing psychotropic drugs and metabolites
   D   the concentration of lithium
   E   regional blood flow

12.2   The following imaging modalities are primarily functional rather than structural imaging techniques:

   A   CT
   B   X-ray radiography
   C   MRS
   D   PET
   E   SPET

12.3   The following imaging techniques require the use of radioactive substances:

   A   CT
   B   MRI
   C ^{31}P-MRS
   D   PET
   E   fMRI

12.4   The following neuroimaging techniques involve the exposure of patients to ionizing radiation:

   A   CT
   B   MRI
   C ^{1}H-MRS
   D   PET
   E   SPECT

12.5 Single-photon emission computerized tomography can be usefully employed to study:

A rCBF changes in migraine
B rCBF changes in auditory hallucinations
C the degree of ventricular enlargement in schizophrenia
D changes over time in cerebral cortical volume in Alzheimer's disease
E the localization of foci of temporal lobe epilepsy

13 NEUROPHYSIOLOGY

Questions

13.1 In the human brain the neuronal resting membrane potential is maintained:

A by the sodium pump
B at around 40–70 mV
C by using ADP for energy
D by active extrusion of potassium ions out of the neurone
E by influx of Ca^{2+}

13.2 In neurones, the action potential:

A spreads by saltatory conduction in unmyelinated fibres
B propagates by the lateral spread of depolarization
C propagates faster in fibres of larger diameter
D is an all-or-none phenomenon
E is triggered by local hyperpolarization

13.3 The following statements concerning synapses and synaptic transmission are true:

A synapses may be found between sensory neurones and sensory receptors
B transmission across electrical synapses is generally slower than across chemical synapses
C EPSPs follow the release of an inhibitory neurotransmitter from the presynaptic neurone
D IPSPs result from depolarization of the post-synaptic membrane
E IPSPs and EPSPs may cancel each other on summation

13.4 Anterior pituitary hormones include:

A prolactin
B antidiuretic hormone
C growth hormone
D thyroxine
E oxytocin

13.5 Hypothalamic release-inhibiting factors include:

A CRF
B somatocrinin
C LH
D MSH release-inhibitory hormone
E dopamine

13.6 The following stages of sleep are correctly paired with their characteristic EEG features:

A stage 0–beta activity
B stage 1–low-voltage theta activity
C stage 2–occasional K complexes
D stage 3–alpha activity
E stage 4–4 to 7 Hz with occasional sleep spindles

13.7 Features of REM sleep include:

A decreased respiratory rate
B the penis is not usually erect in men
C maximal loss of muscle tone
D increased parasympathetic activity
E decreased cerebral blood flow

13.8 Non-REM sleep is associated with:

A decreased heart rate
B upward ocular deviation with few or no eye movements
C noradrenergic neuronal activity in the locus coeruleus in the monoaminergic model of the the sleep–waking cycle
D freedom from dreams
E abolition of tendon reflexes

13.9 The groups of central neurones and their corresponding neurotransmitters that are of importance in the cellular model of the sleep–waking cycle include:

A pontine gigantocellular tegmental fields and dopamine
B caudate nucleus and dopamine
C locus coeruleus and noradrenaline
D dorsal raphe nuclei and serotonin
E laterodorsal tegmental nucleus and acetylcholine

13.10   The following EEG rhythm frequencies are correctly paired with their corresponding EEG classification:

A   3 Hz–alpha
B   11 Hz–beta
C   2 Hz–delta
D   6 Hz–theta
E   8.5 Hz–beta

13.11   The following statements concerning mu and lambda EEG activity are correct:

A   mu activity occurs primarily over the temporal lobes
B   mu activity is related to mnemonic phenomena
C   lambda activity occurs primarily over the prefrontal cortex/frontal eye fields
D   lambda activity is related to ocular movements
E   lambda activity is prominent during REM sleep

13.12   The following statements concerning the EEG are correct:

A   electrodes in conventional EEG recordings are usually positioned according to the International 10-30 System
B   spikes are transient high peaks
C   sphenoidal electrodes are inserted between the mandibular coronoid notch and the zygoma
D   sharp waves last less than 80 ms
E   nasopharyngeal leads can be used to obtain recordings from the medial temporal lobe

13.13   The following drugs are correctly paired with their characteristic effects on the EEG at therapeutic levels:

A   amitriptyline–decreased delta activity
B   lithium–increased alpha activity
C   chlorpromazine–increased beta activity
D   diazepam–decreased beta activity
E   barbiturates–increased alpha activity

14 NEUROCHEMISTRY

Questions

14.1 Central nervous system neurotransmitters include:

A CCK 28
B galanin
C POMC
D ACh
E NO

14.2 Central neuropeptide transmitters include:

A ACTH
B met-enkephalin
C glycine
D dopamine
E dynorphin A

14.3 Neurotransmitter release from synaptic vesicles:

A requires neuronal Na^+ influx
B requires neuronal K^+ efflux
C is quantal
D takes place by exocytosis
E is controlled by neuronal Ca^{2+} influx

14.4 With respect to neurotransmitter release at synapses, calcium ions influence or regulate:

A vesicular fusion
B tonic depolarization of the presynaptic neurone
C the probability of vesicular transmitter release
D transport of synaptic vesicles to the presynaptic active zone of release
E post-tetanic potentiation

14.5 Glutamate receptors include:

A KA2
B M2
C mGluR2
D NMDAR2
E AMPA

14.6   The primary biosynthetic pathway of noradrenaline includes:

   A tyramine
   B COMT
   C dopamine
   D MHPG
   E DOPA

14.7   The catabolic pathway of noradrenaline that starts with the action of COMT includes:

   A 3-methoxy-4-hydroxymandelic acid
   B 3,4-dihydroxymandelic acid
   C DOPAC
   D normetanephrine
   E HVA

14.8   The primary biosynthetic pathway of 5-HT includes:

   A tryptophan hydroxylase
   B 5-HIAA
   C 5-hydroxytryptophan decarboxylase
   D MAO type A
   E 5-deoxytryptophan

14.9   The main catabolic pathway of dopamine that starts with MAO includes:

   A DOPA
   B aldehyde dehydrogenase
   C 3,4-dihydroxyphenylacetaldehyde
   D COMT
   E homovanillic acid

14.10 GABA:

   A is mainly biosynthesized via the action of GABA-T
   B type A receptors act primarily via G protein coupling
   C type B receptor stimulation leads to an increase in chloride ion flow via a receptor-gated ion channel
   D is derived from glutamic acid
   E is catabolized to glutamic acid

14.11   Acetylcholine:

   A   has a strong affinity for nicotinic receptors
   B   is derived from acetyl CoA and choline
   C   is biosynthesized in a reaction involving cholinesterase
   D   is catabolized mainly to acetyl CoA and choline
   E   is catabolized mainly by hydrolysis

15 General Principles of Psychopharmacology

Questions

15.1   The following drugs are correctly paired with the names of those involved in their initial synthesis:

   A   chlorpromazine–Charpentier
   B   haloperidol–Lundbeck
   C   lithium–Kline
   D   clozapine–Laborit
   E   chlordiazepoxide–Sternbach

15.2   The following psychotropic drugs are correctly paired with the names of those involved in their development:

   A   MAOIs–Kline
   B   imipramine–Kuhn
   C   lithium–Cade
   D   chlorpromazine–Delay and Deniker
   E   clozapine–Kane

15.3   The following psychotropic drugs are correctly paired with the decade in which their introduction into clinical psychiatric use first took place:

   A   MAOIs–1960s
   B   SSRIs–1990s
   C   lithium–1940s
   D   chlorpromazine–1950s
   E   barbiturates–1960s

15.4   The following antipsychotic drugs are correctly classified in the groups to which they belong:

   A   perphenazine–aliphatic phenothiazine
   B   procyclidine–anticholinergic
   C   pimozide–diphenylbutylpiperidine
   D   thioridazine–thioxanthene
   E   haloperidol–butyrophenone

15.5 Antimuscarinic drugs that may be used in the treatment of parkinsonism resulting from pharmacotherapy with antipsychotics include:

A amperozide
B methixene
C orphenadrine
D biperiden
E pericyazine

15.6 Antidepressants that act by inhibiting MAO include:

A isocarboxazid
B maprotiline
C nefazodone
D tranylcypromine
E moclobemide

16 PHARMACOKINETICS

Questions

16.1 Parenteral routes that may be used for drug administration include:

A sublingual
B buccal
C inhalational
D subcutaneous
E topical

16.2 The rate of absorption of drugs administered intramuscularly is increased in the following circumstances:

A for drugs that are more lipid-soluble
B for drugs with a higher relative molecular mass
C during emotional excitement
D in cardiac failure
E immediately following physical exercise

16.3 An increased or relatively high volume of distribution for a drug is generally associated with:

A increased lipid solubility of the drug
B weight gain
C younger age
D longer duration of drug action
E drugs that are highly protein bound

16.4 Plasma protein binding is:

A generally irreversible
B mainly to α_1-acid glycoprotein for drugs that are acidic
C usually increased following surgery
D decreased in hepatic disease
E competitive

16.5   The blood–brain barrier is:

    A   partly composed of a gliovascular membrane
    B   partly composed of Purkinje cells
    C   impermeable to most psychotropic drugs
    D   crossed by lithium ions by diffusion
    E   crossed by levodopa by diffusion

16.6   Hepatic phase I biotransformation:

    A   plays an important part in the metabolism of many antidepressants
    B   plays an important part in the metabolism of lithium
    C   can involve the cytochrome P450 system
    D   can involve synthetic conjugation reactions
    E   contributes to the first-pass effect

17 PHARMACODYNAMICS

Questions

17.1   Clozapine has a higher potency of action than do, in general, typical antipsychotics on the following receptors:

A   D1
B   D4
C   5-HT$_2$
D   α-adrenergic
E   muscarinic

17.2   Side-effects of chlorpromazine resulting from antidopaminergic actions include:

A   akathisia
B   pyrexia
C   gynaecomastia
D   postural hypotension
E   ejaculatory failure

17.3   In the central nervous system, monoamine oxidase type A acts on:

A   noradrenaline
B   serotonin
C   dopamine
D   tyramine
E   phenylethylamine

17.4   Effects of chronic lithium treatment include:

A   decreased erythrocyte choline levels
B   increased Na,K-ATPase pump activity
C   increased serotonergic neurotransmission
D   increased erythrocyte phospholipid catabolism
E   decreased central dopamine synthesis

17.5   Peripheral antimuscarinic side-effects of tricyclic antidepressants include:

A   blurred vision
B   weight gain
C   constipation
D   vomiting
E   urinary retention

17.6 Binding to $GABA_A$ receptors is the important postulated mode of action in the brain for the anxiolytic and/or sedative-hypnotic actions of:

  A diazepam
  B buspirone
  C propranolol
  D zopiclone
  E zolpidem

17.7 The following are antiepileptic drugs that are believed to achieve their anticonvulsant action primarily by acting on the GABAergic system:

  A sodium valproate
  B gabapentin
  C vigabatrin
  D lamotrigine
  E tiagabine

17.8 Electroconvulsive therapy causes an acute increase in the activity of the following neurotransmitters in the brain:

  A noradrenaline
  B serotonin
  C dopamine
  D acetylcholine
  E GABA

18 ADVERSE DRUG REACTIONS

Questions

18.1   The following features suggest that an adverse drug reaction is caused by an allergic reaction to the drug:

    A the time-course of the reaction closely mirrors that of the pharmacodynamic action

    B the adverse drug reaction manifests only after repeated drug exposure

    C there is a dose-related effect

    D the adverse drug reaction only occurs with therapeutic or higher doses

    E a hypersensitivity reaction occurs that is unrelated to the pharmacological actions of the drug

18.2   Types of allergic reaction to drugs involving II, III or IV hypersensitivity reactions include:

    A anaphylactic shock

    B haemolytic anaemia

    C thrombocytopenia

    D drug displacement from binding sites

    E allergic liver damage

18.3   Characteristic features of neuroleptic malignant syndrome include:

    A hyperthermia

    B tachycardia

    C leucopenia

    D muscle flaccidity

    E fluctuating level of consciousness

18.4   Long-term high-dose pharmacotherapy with chlorpromazine may lead to purplish pigmentation of the:

    A skin

    B CSF

    C conjunctiva

    D cornea

    E retina

18.5 Recognized sensitivity reactions caused by typical antipsychotics (neuroleptics) include:

A hypothermia
B haemolytic anaemia
C agranulocytosis
D leucopenia
E leucocytosis

18.6 Side-effects of clozapine include:

A neutropenia
B agranulocytosis
C pyrexia
D jaundice
E hypersalivation

18.7 Effects of antimuscarinic drugs used in parkinsonism include:

A blurred vision
B improvement of tardive dyskinesia
C excitement
D gastrointestinal disturbances
E sialorrhoea

18.8 The therapeutic index is:

A directly proportional to the therapeutic dose of the drug
B directly proportional to the toxic dose of the drug
C low for lithium
D low for diazepam
E low for amitriptyline

18.9 Side-effects of lithium in its therapeutic range include:

A oedema
B oliguria
C metallic taste
D coarse tremor
E dry mouth

18.10   Signs of lithium intoxication include:

A   lack of coordination
B   blurred vision
C   dysarthria
D   hyperreflexia of the limbs
E   tinnitus

18.11   Long-term treatment with lithium may give rise to:

A   goitre
B   nephrotoxicity
C   T-wave flattening on the ECG
D   cardiac arrhythmias
E   memory impairment

18.12   Side-effects of tricyclic antidepressants include:

A   photosensitization
B   testicular atrophy
C   black tongue
D   postural hypotension
E   eosinophilia

18.13   Foods to avoid while being treated with a monoamine oxidase inhibitor include:

A   caviar
B   cottage cheese
C   pickled herring
D   yeast extract
E   milk

18.14   Drugs that interact dangerously with monoamine oxidase inhibitors include:

A   propranolol
B   fenfluramine
C   ephedrine
D   diazepam
E   clomipramine

18.15   Diazepam can lead to:

A   psychomotor impairment
B   headache
C   respiratory stimulation
D   dry mouth
E   a withdrawal syndrome

18.16   For a patient regularly taking disulfiram at a therapeutic dosage, the ingestion of alcohol:

   A   causes unpleasant side-effects as a result of the accumulation of formaldehyde
   B   often causes tachycardia
   C   often causes severe hypertension
   D   in large amounts can lead to cardiac arrhythmias
   E   in large amounts can lead to air hunger

18.17   In men, side-effects of cyproterone acetate include:

   A   gynaecomastia
   B   acne vulgaris
   C   weight loss
   D   increased energy
   E   female pattern of pubic hair growth

19 GENETICS

Questions

19.1 Meiosis:

    A involves one stage of cell division
    B involves chromosomal double division
    C results in haploid cells
    D includes the stage of interphase during which recombination takes place
    E occurs in gametogenesis

19.2 The following statements concerning normal gene structure in humans are correct:

    A amino acids are coded for by introns
    B amino acids are coded for by codons
    C the 3' end is upstream
    D the 3' end contains a poly A addition site
    E there is an upstream site regulating transcription

19.3 Karyotyping involves:

    A dispersion
    B fixation
    C transcription
    D translation
    E Southern blotting

19.4 Transcription involves:

    A tRNA
    B ultimately the creation of an mRNA template based on the exons and introns of DNA
    C disomy
    D the creation of a primary RNA transcript
    E peptide synthesis

19.5 The following patterns of inheritance are correctly paired with some of their characteristic features:

    A Mendel's first law–independent assortment
    B autosomal dominant inheritance–horizontal transmission
    C autosomal recessive inheritance–heterozygotes are generally carriers
    D X-linked recessive inheritance–male heterozygotes are generally carriers
    E X-linked dominant inheritance–male-to-male transmission does not occur

19.6 Genetic markers can be used in:

A linkage analysis
B genomic imprinting
C prenatal diagnosis
D presymptomatic diagnosis
E restriction endonuclease synthesis

19.7 In molecular genetics, the lod score:

A is calculated by taking the natural logarithm of the ratio of two probabilities
B involves the probability of there being linkage
C involves the probability of there being no measurable linkage
D is the maximum likelihood score of the ratio of linkage to no linkage
E is a measure of the probability of two genetic loci being linked

19.8 Down's syndrome may result from:

A non-disjunction during meiosis
B exchange of genetic material between chromosome 21 and chromosome 13
C exchange of genetic material between chromosome 21 and chromosome 21
D trisomy 17
E mosaicism

19.9 The following disorders are correctly paired with their genotypes:

A Edward's syndrome–47, +19
B Patau's syndrome–47, +13
C cri-du-chat syndrome–47, +5
D triple X syndrome–48, XXXY
E Turner's syndrome–45, X

19.10 Autosomal dominant disorders include:

A Tay–Sachs disease
B galactosaemia
C Huntington's disease
D tuberous sclerosis
E neurofibromatosis

19.11 Autosomal recessive disorders of protein metabolism include:

A cystinuria
B citrullinaemia
C maple syrup urine disease
D von Hippel–Lindau syndrome
E Hurler syndrome

19.12   Autosomal recessive disorders of carbohydrate metabolism include:

    A Niemann–Pick disease
    B Hunter syndrome
    C Pompe disease
    D Wilson disease
    E hereditary fructose intolerance

19.13   X-linked recessive disorders include:

    A Lesch–Nyan syndrome
    B fragile X syndrome
    C Lowe syndrome
    D Rett syndrome
    E testicular feminization syndrome

20 Epidemiology

Questions

20.1 Types of prevalence include:

A point
B population at risk
C lifetime
D disease rate at post mortem
E birth defect rate

20.2 The incidence of a disease:

A can be expressed in units such as 'per 1000' or 'per 100 000'
B includes the morbidity rate
C includes the mortality rate
D is inversely proportional to the prevalence in the steady state
E is calculated by a formula that includes individuals who have already had the disease

20.3 The following measures do not have any units:

A prevalence
B chronicity
C relative risk
D odds ratio
E SMR

20.4 Important confounders that sometimes, though not always, need to be taken into account in determining the mortality rate from a disease include:

A gender
B population size
C age
D ethnicity
E age-standardized mortality rate

20.5   A relative risk for a disease:

A   if zero, is the null hypothesis in hypothesis testing
B   if 0.5 and significantly different to the null hypothesis value, is evidence of a positive association between the disease and the relative risk factor
C   may be calculated in prospective epidemiological studies
D   with respect to a given risk factor is the ratio of the incidence of the disease in people exposed to that risk factor to the incidence of the disease in people not exposed to the same risk factor
E   that strongly suggests an association between the disease and the risk factor does not necessary imply a causative or preventative role for the risk factor

20.6   In an epidemiological study, of those exposed to a given risk factor, let the number with the disease be *a* and without the disease be *b*. For those not exposed to the risk factor, let the number with the disease be *c* and without the disease be *d*. The following statements are correct:

A   the incidence of the disease in people exposed to the risk factor is $a/(a+b)$
B   the relative risk is $c(a+b)/[a(c+d)]$
C   the total number with no disease is $b+d$
D   the odds ratio is $bc/(ad)$
E   the attributable risk is $a/(a+b) - c/(c+d)$

20.7   Sources of information for determining the morbidity rate of a disease include:

A   hospitals
B   general practices
C   records of death registration
D   case registers
E   questionnaires

20.8   The PSE:

A   is a self-rated questionnaire
B   can be used with CATEGO
C   has a good reliability for the diagnosis of schizophrenia
D   has a good reliability for the diagnosis of personality disorder
E   can be used via the ID to determine caseness

20.9   The GHQ:

A   consists of 60 items
B   is observer rated
C   was devised by Wing
D   is particularly useful in identifying psychotic cases
E   is particularly useful in the assessment of anxiety and depression in outpatient and primary care medical patients

20.10   In a generalized set of diagnostic and test results, let the number of individuals that are respectively true positive, false positive, false negative and true negative be a, b, c and d. The following statements are true:

   A   the sensitivity of the test is a/c
   B   the specificity of the test is $d/(a + c)$
   C   the predictive value of a positive test result is $a/(a + b)$
   D   the predictive value of a negative test result is $d/(c + d)$
   E   the efficiency of the test is $a/(a + b + c + d)$

21 Medical Ethics and Principles of Law

Questions

Note that many of the questions in this chapter refer in particular to British law.

21.1   Under British Social Security Regulations, an appointee:

    A has the power to deal with the claimant's capital
    B has the power to receive any benefits payable to the claimant
    C must be aged 21 years or over
    D can exercise any rights and duties that the claimant has under the Social Security Acts and Regulations
    E can have his or her appointment revoked at any time by the Secretary of State

21.2   The following statements concerning a power of attorney are true:

    A it involves the donor giving legal authority to an advocate to manage their affairs
    B the donor has sole responsibility in the decision as to whether power of attorney is given provided they fully understand the implications of what they are undertaking
    C if the donor loses their mental capacity to manage their own affairs then an ordinary power of attorney must ensure that the financial needs of the donor and their family are adequately met
    D regulation of an enduring power of attorney occurs via a local magistrate
    E an ordinary power of attorney does not have to allow the donor's financial affairs to be dealt with generally, but can be limited to specific matters

21.3   The following statements are correct:

    A 'testamentary capacity' refers to the competence of a mentally ill person to give evidence on oath
    B a plea of 'diminished responsibility' can only be entered in murder cases
    C the Court of Protection is an office of the Supreme Court
    D the Court of Protection has the power to determine how patients placed under its care shall be treated
    E a valid will is automatically invalidated by subsequent loss of a 'sound disposing mind'

21.4   The following statements concerning the Court of Protection are correct:

    A applications can only be made on behalf of patients suffering from dementia
    B the person appointed to manage the patient's affairs is known as the receiver
    C in order to avoid a conflict of interest, the person appointed to manage the patient's affairs must not be a relative or friend
    D the medical recommendation must be by a doctor approved under the Mental Health Act
    E the patient has the right to object to the application

21.5   The following statements concerning driving in Britain are correct:

A the responsibility for making the decision about whether or not psychiatric patients should continue to drive is that of their doctor

B drivers are not obliged to keep the DVLA informed of any condition that may impair their ability to drive

C a patient's doctor is responsible for advising the patient to inform the DVLA of a condition likely to make driving dangerous

D Group 1 licences are not available to patients with a Mobility Allowance

E both Group 1 and Group 2 licences may be restricted to a shorter duration for medical reasons

21.6   The DVLA advises that psychiatric patients should not drive motor cars or motor bikes in Britain for at least 6 months after:

A an anxiety state

B an episode of dysthmia

C an acute schizophrenic psychotic episode requiring hospital admission

D a hypomanic episode requiring hospital admission

E a diagnosis being made of severe mental handicap

21.7   After an acute psychotic episode requiring hospital admission, the criteria that must be met during the following 3 years in order to be granted British Group 2 driving entitlement include:

A the patient's condition must be stable

B the patient must be symptom free

C the patient must not be on treatment with large doses of antipsychotics

D the patient must not be on treatment with lithium

E the patient must be examined by a consultant psychiatrist

21.8   Regular use of, or dependency on, the following substances, confirmed by medical enquiry, will lead in Britain to Group 1 entitlement driving licence revocation or refusal for at least a 6-month period:

A cannabis

B ecstacy

C LSD

D benzodiazepines

E cocaine

Questions

Note that the questions in this chapter refer to the Mental Health Act 1983 of England and Wales.

22.1 Under the Mental Health Act 1983:

   A a parent usually takes preference over an adult son or daughter in determining the nearest relative
   B the term 'patient' is defined as a person suffering or appearing to be suffering from mental disorder
   C the term 'mental illness' is defined as mental disorder, arrested or incomplete development of mind, or psychopathic disorder
   D rehabilitation under medical supervision is not included in the term 'medical treatment'
   E both 'mental impairment' and 'severe mental impairment' are defined

22.2 A person may be dealt with under the Mental Health Act 1983 as suffering from mental disorder by reason only of manifesting:

   A sexual deviancy
   B alcohol dependence
   C suicidal behaviour
   D promiscuity
   E dependence on cocaine

22.3 Under the Mental Health Act 1983, a guardianship application:

   A requires one written medical recommendation from a doctor who is approved under the Mental Health Act
   B requires that the patient be at least 14 years of age
   C requires that the guardian be a local social services authority
   D after approval, does not confer on the guardian the power to specify the place of residence of the patient
   E may be made only by an approved social worker

22.4 The following civil treatment orders are correctly paired with the corresponding Sections of the Mental Health Act 1983:

   A emergency admission for assessment–Section 4
   B nurses holding power of voluntary inpatient–Section 5(4)
   C interim hospital order–Section 37
   D admission by police–Section 135
   E power of entry to home and removal to place of safety–Section 136

22.5 Psychiatric treatments that can be administered under Section 57 of the Mental Health Act 1983 include:

A leucotomy
B hormone implantation
C castration
D ECT
E an orally administered antidepressant at a therapeutic dose

22.6 The following forensic treatment orders for mentally abnormal offenders are correctly paired with the corresponding Sections of the Mental Health Act 1983:

A remand to hospital for treatment–Section 36
B restriction order–Section 41
C remand to hospital for report–Section 49
D transfer of a sentenced prisoner to hospital–Section 47
E urgent transfer to hospital of a remand prisoner–Section 48

22.7 Under the Mental Health Act 1983, an approved social worker may make an application for:

A Section 2
B Section 4
C Section 5(2)
D Section 41
E Section 136

22.8 The medical recommendations for the following Sections of the Mental Health Act 1983 require that, in the case when one doctor is required, he or she is approved under Section 12 of the Mental Health Act, and in the case when more than one doctor is required, that at least one of the doctors is similarly approved:

A Section 3
B Section 4
C Section 35
D Section 36
E Section 47

22.9 The following Sections of the Mental Health Act 1983 are correctly paired with their corresponding maximum durations (without renewal):

A Section 3–28 days
B Section 5(4)–72 hours
C Section 135–28 days
D Section 35–6 months
E Section 36–6 months

22.10   Patients detained under Section 2 of the Mental Health Act 1983 may be discharged
        by:

        A   the hospital managers
        B   the approved social worker involved in their admission
        C   their nearest relative
        D   their RMO
        E   a MHRT

23 CLASSIFICATION

Questions

23.1 Mood (affective) disorders in ICD-10 include the following major categories:

A manic episode
B major depression
C persistent mood [affective] disorders
D unspecified non-organic psychosis
E bipolar affective disorder

23.2 Types of schizophrenia that are classified in ICD-10 under F20 Schizophrenia include:

A disorganized
B paranoid
C residual
D undifferentiated
E simple

23.3 The following types of problem are correctly paired with the axes of DSM-IV under which they are measured:

A general medical conditions–axis I
B mental retardation–axis III
C psychosocial problems–axis V
D personality disorders–axis II
E clinical disorders–axis IV

23.4 Names of types of personality disorder classified in DSM-IV include:

A anxious
B dependent
C anankastic
D borderline
E paranoid

24 Physical Therapies

Questions

This chapter does not consider pharmacotherapy, which is covered in Chapters 15–18.

24.1 Individuals who played a key role in the development of ECT in the twentieth century include:

 A Bini
 B Meduna
 C Kane
 D Cerletti
 E Charcot

24.2 Indications for ECT include:

 A puerperal depressive illness
 B mild depressive illness
 C mania
 D catatonic schizophrenia
 E simple phobias

24.3 The role of atropine administered during ECT is to reduce:

 A violent movements
 B damage from biting
 C muscarinic actions of another drug given
 D memory impairment
 E secretions

24.4 The clinical indications for sleep deprivation in mood disorders include:

 A as an aid to diagnosis
 B as an antidepressant in treatment-resistant patients
 C to augment the response to antidepressants
 D to treat SAD
 E to hasten the onset of action of lithium

24.5 Individuals involved in the development of psychosurgery include:

 A Jacobsen
 B Kretschmer
 C Fulton
 D Moniz
 E Burckhardt

24.6   In British psychiatry, psychosurgery may be considered as a last-resort treatment in:

    A   depression
    B   bulimia nervosa
    C   paedophilia
    D   obsessive–compulsive disorder
    E   anxiety states

24.7   Current methods for making psychosurgical stereotaxic lesions that are used in Britain and the USA include:

    A   proton laser ablation
    B   the gamma knife
    C   electrocautery
    D   radioactive yttrium implantation
    E   thermocoagulation

24.8   Psychosurgical operations in current use include:

    A   optic tractotomy
    B   subcaudate tractotomy
    C   cingulotomy
    D   limbic leucotomy
    E   capsulotomy

25 Organic Psychiatry

Questions

25.1   Causes of dementia include:

    A multiple sclerosis
    B normal-pressure hydrocephalus
    C hypoparathyroidism
    D caffeine
    E vitamin D deficiency

25.2   Systemic disorders that may cause organic mood disorder include:

    A SLE
    B pernicious anaemia
    C rheumatoid arthritis
    D neoplasia
    E carcinoid syndrome

25.3   Common symptoms of anxiety that can be secondary to hyperventilation include:

    A constipation
    B reduced frequency of micturition
    C chest pain
    D paraesthesia
    E choking

25.4   Causes of organic personality disorder include:

    A clozapine
    B γ-linolenic acid
    C hepatolenticular degeneration
    D corticosteroids
    E Huntington's disease

26 PSYCHOACTIVE SUBSTANCE-USE DISORDERS

Questions

26.1 The following statements concerning acute intoxication are correct:

A its intensity is not dose related
B it may result in disturbed perception
C it may result in disturbed affect
D recovery is usually incomplete
E the effects often continue for at least several weeks after the episode has stopped

26.2 The following features caused by psychoactive substances are correctly paired with clinical conditions in which they can occur:

A compulsion to take the substance–dependence syndrome
B adverse social consequences–harmful use
C LSD-induced sudden aggressive behaviour–pathological intoxication
D confabulation–amnesic syndrome
E hallucinations–delirium tremens

26.3 Residual and late-onset psychotic disorder, caused by psychoactive substance use, is subdivided into the following diagnoses in ICD-10:

A withdrawal state
B Korsakov's psychosis
C personality or behaviour disorder
D dementia
E flashbacks

26.4 The following represent approximately 1 unit of alcohol:

A a bottle of wine
B a glass of sherry
C a single measure of whisky
D 4 g of ethanol
E one pint of standard-strength beer

26.5 Physical effects that may be caused by excessive alcohol intake include:

A vitamin C deficiency
B holiday heart syndrome
C hepatitis
D gonadal atrophy
E pseudo-Cushing's syndrome

26.6   Features of fetal alcohol syndrome include:

   A   absent philtrum
   B   macrocephaly
   C   high-set ears
   D   ocular hypertelorism
   E   strabismus

26.7   Characteristic features of Wernicke's encephalopathy include:

   A   nystagmus
   B   petechial haemorrhages in the mammillary bodies
   C   flapping tremor of the hands
   D   ataxia
   E   clouding of consciousness

26.8   Wernicke's encephalopathy is a recognized complication of:

   A   carcinoma of the stomach
   B   chronic alcoholism
   C   persistent vomiting
   D   viral infection
   E   starvation

26.9   In delirium tremens:

   A   the mortality is around 25%
   B   the drug of choice in its treatment is paraldehyde
   C   nursing is best carried out in a room that is as dark as possible
   D   pyrexia is a common finding
   E   the EEG typically shows excess slow activity

26.10   In Britain, the following drugs require a special licence to be prescribed in the treatment of drug addiction:

   A   heroin
   B   methadone
   C   cannabis
   D   LSD
   E   cocaine

26.11 In Britain, under the Misuse of Drugs Act 1971, the following orally administered substances are classified as class A drugs:

A codeine
B amphetamines
C barbiturates
D meprobamate
E cannabis

26.12 The majority of opiate addicts in the UK are:

A introduced to the drug by a doctor
B women
C members of ethnic minorities
D members of medical or allied professions
E aged under 20 years

26.13 Characteristic features of chronic opioid dependence include:

A mydriasis
B increased sexual activity in men
C diarrhoea
D tremor
E malaise

26.14 Acute effects of LSD ingestion commonly include:

A clouding of consciousness
B mydriasis
C reduced tendon reflexes
D synaesthesia
E auditory hallucinations

26.15 Tetrahydrocannabinols:

A are responsible for most of the psychological effects of cannabis
B are strongly lipophobic
C cannot be detected in the blood
D can cause decreased hippocampal neuronal density
E have anticholinergic effects

Questions

27.1   Historical contributions in the field of mental illness include:

A   Kurt Schneider's attribution of negative symptoms to neuronal loss
B   Bleuler's attribution of secondary status to delusions and hallucinations in schizophrenia
C   Kraepelin's introduction of the term 'schizophrenia'
D   the influence of the writings of Sigmund Freud on Kraepelin's concept of schizophrenia
E   Bleuler's attribution of secondary status to symptoms of ambivalence, autism, affective incongruity and disturbance of association of thought

27.2   The following are Schneiderian first-rank symptoms of schizophrenia:

A   incongruity of affect
B   Gedankenlautwerden
C   delusional perception
D   auditory hallucinations in the second person
E   perplexity

27.3   In the ICD-10 classification of schizophrenia:

A   little weight is given to the presence of Schneiderian first-rank symptoms
B   it is not possible to diagnose schizophrenia in the absence of Schneiderian first-rank symptoms
C   symptoms should have been present for a duration of one month or more in order to diagnose the hebephrenic subtype
D   a diagnosis of schizoaffective disorder is made if affective symptoms are also present
E   the diagnosis of simple schizophrenia requires past evidence of at least one schizophrenic episode with positive symptoms, and a period of at least a year in which the frequency of positive symptoms has been minimal, and negative symptoms present

27.4   In hebephrenic schizophrenia:

A   the age of onset is generally earlier than in paranoid schizophrenia
B   there are few affective symptoms
C   the prognosis is generally good
D   delusions tend to be well systematized
E   mannerisms are common

27.5   The following statements considering Liddle's syndromes of symptoms in schizophrenia are true:

   A   the psychomotor poverty syndrome is characterized by poverty of speech, flatness of affect and decreased spontaneous movement
   B   the reality distortion syndrome is characterized by disorder of the form of thought
   C   the psychomotor poverty syndrome is associated with hypoperfusion of the left dorsal prefrontal cortex
   D   the disorganization syndrome is associated with hypoperfusion of the right ventral prefrontal cortex
   E   hypofrontality in schizophrenia is more often seen in those with an acute florid illness

27.6   The following statements concerning the epidemiology of schizophrenia are true:

   A   the incidence of schizophrenia is equal in all socioeconomic classes
   B   the prevalence is higher in rural than in urban areas, and this can be attributed to 'social drift'
   C   the poorer prognosis in men than in women may be partly explained by the later onset of schizophrenia in men than in women
   D   the incidence of schizophrenia is approximately 1%
   E   the point prevalence of schizophrenia is approximately 1%

27.7   In schizophrenia:

   A   when both parents are affected, their offspring are almost certain to be affected
   B   the offspring of an unaffected monozygotic co-twin are less likely to be affected than the offspring of the proband
   C   the offspring of an unaffected dizygotic twin are less likely to be affected than the offspring of the proband
   D   adopted-away children of schizophrenic mothers have similar rates of schizophrenia as non-adopted-away children
   E   the mode of inheritance is likely to be a single major locus

27.8   The neurodevelopmental model of schizophrenia accounts for:

   A   the earlier onset in men than in women
   B   the higher concordance rate for monozygotic than for dizygotic twins
   C   the winter excess of births in schizophrenia
   D   the increased relapse rate in those schizophrenic patients who reside with relatives who demonstrate high expressed emotion
   E   the excess of minor physical abnormalities reported in schizophrenia

27.9　Expressed emotion:

A　has an effect on the relapse rates of schizophrenic patients only
B　is assessed using the Camberwell Assessment of Need
C　probably exerts its effect through changes in physiological arousal in the schizophrenic subject
D　may account for the good prognosis seen in schizophrenia in the less developed world
E　if high, can be modified in its effects on the patient by reducing contact with family members to less than 35 hours' contact per week

27.10　In a 19-year-old man, the following support the diagnosis of schizophrenia:

A　auditory hallucinations
B　suicidal thoughts
C　sensitive ideas of reference
D　delusional perception
E　made impulses

27.11　The brains of patients with schizophrenia:

A　show a lower ventricle–brain ratio than do controls
B　are shorter than those of controls
C　have larger lateral ventricles on average compared with controls
D　can be indistinguishable from normal controls
E　are more likely to be abnormal in men

27.12　Atypical antipsychotic drugs:

A　do not produce catalepsy in animals
B　are the treatment of choice in a violent acutely psychotic patient
C　have a reduced potential for extra pyramidal side-effects
D　have a reduced potential for side-effects
E　do not elevate prolactin levels in man

27.13　In the treatment of schizophrenia:

A　around 10% of patients are likely to be non-compliant with prescribed oral medication
B　using depot neuroleptic medication does not alter relapse rates
C　there is no role for the use of electroconvulsive therapy
D　psychoeducational family programmes are successful in reducing the risk of relapse
E　extrapyramidal side-effects occur in up to 10% of patients taking conventional neuroleptic medication

27.14   The following features in a psychotic individual suggest that schizophrenia is not the primary diagnosis:

    A delusional mood
    B clouding of consciousness
    C écho de la pensée
    D Lilliputian visual hallucinations
    E twilight state

27.15   The following are poor prognostic features of schizophrenia:

    A sudden onset
    B later onset
    C family history of affective disorder
    D ventricular enlargement
    E positive symptoms

27.16   The following statements are true:

    A the Fregoli syndrome is a rare delusional disorder in which the patient believes that a familiar person has taken on different appearances
    B the Capgras' syndrome has been described with reference to inanimate objects as well as people
    C Cotard's syndrome is also called erotomania
    D the object of attention in a case of Othello syndrome can safely be reassured
    E in Cotard's syndrome the patient may believe that they do not exist

27.17   The following statements with regard to schizoaffective disorder are true:

    A the prognosis is the same for both manic and depressive subtypes
    B the concept was first introduced by Kasanin in 1933
    C it is used to describe a schizophrenic patient who demonstrates depressive symptoms
    D the prognosis lies between that of mood disorders and that of schizophrenia
    E continuum theorists, e.g. Kendall, would consider it to be an illness distinct from schizophrenia and affective disorder

27.18   A schizophrenia-like psychosis is seen in:

    A Wilson's disease
    B alcohol dependency
    C heroin dependency
    D epilepsy
    E Behçet's disease

27.19   In schizophrenia, brain CT scan changes are associated with:

A   good premorbid adjustment
B   negative symptoms
C   a negative family history of schizophrenia
D   reduced parahippocampal volume
E   disorientation for age

27.20   Patients with schizophrenia who are being discharged from hospital to home:

A   are all subject to Section 117 aftercare
B   are subject to the Care Programme Approach
C   should generally be advised to remain on antipsychotic medication for a minimum of a year
D   should be advised to notify the DVLA if they have just experienced an acute psychotic episode
E   are as likely to remain well on oral medication as on depot medication

Questions

28.1   In the ICD-10 description of bipolar affective disorder:

A it is possible to experience delusions while hypomanic
B a symptom duration of one month is required for the diagnosis of a depressive episode
C repeated episodes of mania without depression are classified as bipolar
D manic episodes tend to last longer than depressive episodes
E it is possible for depressive and manic symptoms to alternate every hour

28.2   The Newcastle school of thought would consider that the following are suggestive of an endogenous rather than a reactive form of depression:

A initial insomnia
B anhedonia
C depressive thought content
D diurnal variation of mood
E psychomotor agitation

28.3   Bipolar depression, compared with unipolar depression:

A is more common in women
B has a similar age of onset
C is more likely show a seasonal pattern of mood variation
D is distinguishable on the basis of a sleep EEG
E is likely to result in a greater number of episodes

28.4   The following statements are true:

A 'double depression' refers to a particularly severe depressive episode
B patients in depressive stupor are unlikely to later recall events that took place at the time
C symptoms must be present for at least two years for a diagnosis of dysthymia
D rapid cycling of mood in bipolar disorder predicts a poorer prognosis
E it is possible to be suffering from depression without being aware of feeling depressed

28.5   Grief:

  A has four phases
  B may result in autonomic symptoms
  C typically lasts about 6 weeks
  D results after several weeks in the phase of acceptance and adjustment
  E is more likely to be abnormal if the subject had mixed feelings towards the deceased

28.6   The following statements considering the epidemiology of depression are true:

  A the incidence of severe depressive symptoms is higher in middle-class than in working-class women
  B bipolar mood disorder is commoner in the upper social classes
  C the lifetime risk of suffering from depressive episodes in Western countries is higher in women than in men
  D the average age of onset is earlier in bipolar disorder than in unipolar depression
  E those who are not married appear to be protected to some extent from developing depression

28.7   In affective disorder, the following statements are true:

  A in bipolar probands there is an increased risk of bipolar disorder in first-degree relatives, but no increase in unipolar depression in the relatives compared with the general population
  B in unipolar probands there is an increased risk of unipolar disorder in first-degree relatives, but no increase in bipolar depression in the relatives compared with the general population
  C the monozygotic–dizygotic concordance rates indicate that bipolar disorder is more influenced by genetic factors than unipolar disorder
  D linkage studies are straightforward and likely to yield results
  E adopting away the child of a bipolar patient has little effect upon the chances of the child later developing bipolar disorder itself

28.8   The following features are seen in severe depressive illness:

  A poverty of thought
  B guilt about actual misdemeanours
  C subjective complaints of poor memory
  D excessive sleeping
  E indecisiveness

28.9 The following features in an apparently depressed individual suggest that an affective disorder is not the primary diagnosis:

A derogatory auditory hallucinations in the second person
B a conviction that one is dead and rotting
C auditory hallucinations commenting on one's actions
D a conviction that ones' actions are being controlled by Satan
E irritability

28.10 The following statements with regard to the management of affective disorder are true:

A if the family show high expressed emotion, limiting contact to less than 35 hours per week improves the patient's prognosis
B after the initial treatment achieves a response, it is appropriate to reduce the dose of antidepressant to a lower maintenance dose
C electroconvulsive therapy can be used in the treatment of resistant mania
D sudden withdrawal of lithium is best avoided
E antidepressants are the best treatment for delusional depression

28.11 The following are recognized as causes of severe depression:

A hypothyroidism
B Pick's disease
C brucellosis
D Cushing's syndrome
E cerebral infarct

28.12 There is an increased risk of suicide in:

A women
B times of war
C men following bereavement of spouse
D paranoid schizophrenia recently recovered
E those with personality disorder

Questions

29.1 In neurotic disorders:

  A there is an excess in men in childhood
  B psychoanalytic psychotherapy is usually the treatment of choice
  C there is an excess of deaths due to circulatory disease
  D diazepam is more efficacious than dothiepin
  E Freud suggested that repression of the death instinct (thanatos) generates anxiety resulting in symptom formation

29.2 In defining fear as phobic, the following statements pertain:

  A it leads to avoidant behaviour
  B it always results in a panic attack
  C it is in proportion to objective risk as explained by Seligman's preparedness
  D it is generalized
  E it is beyond voluntary control

29.3 The following statements considering phobic anxiety disorders are true:

  A social phobia is commoner in men
  B anticipatory anxiety follows exposure to the feared situation or object
  C phobias are more likely to arise in response to snakes than to guns
  D the prognosis in specific phobia is worse the earlier the onset
  E benzodiazepines used in conjunction with exposure therapy improve the response rate compared with exposure therapy alone

29.4 In generalized anxiety disorder:

  A the diagnostic reliability is high
  B onset is generally later than for other anxiety disorders
  C environmental factors play a larger part in the aetiology than in panic disorder
  D uncontrollable worry is a commonly reported symptom
  E there is autonomic overactivity

29.5 Obsessional symptoms:

A can often be pleasurable
B must be present for at least 6 months in order to qualify for an ICD-10 diagnosis of obsessive–compulsive disorder
C are thought by psychoanalysts to arise from the defence mechanisms of displacement, undoing and reaction formation
D arising in the presence of Tourette's syndrome are regarded as part of Tourette's syndrome
E when arising in the presence of schizophrenia are regarded as two separate concurrently occurring conditions

29.6 Patients with obsessive–compulsive disorder:

A are believed by psychoanalysts to have regressed to the oral stage of development
B show increased blood flow to the caudate nucleus on functional neuroimaging
C are as likely to benefit from treatment with maprotiline as from treatment with clomipramine
D usually relapse after stopping antidepressant therapy
E have a better outlook if they demonstrate symptoms involving symmetry

29.7 The following features in a patient complaining of anxiety would increase the likelihood of a diagnosis of panic disorder:

A duration of up to 12 hours
B feeling worried all the time
C feeling of imminent death
D phobic avoidance of crowds
E abrupt onset

29.8 The following features favour a neurosis rather than a psychosis:

A coherent speech
B panic attacks
C incongruity of affect
D open public defaecation
E synaesthesia

29.9   The following statements with regard to post-traumatic stress disorder (PTSD) are true:

    A there is evidence that opioid function may be disturbed
    B viewing the dead body of a relative after a disaster increases the risk
    C drug therapy is ineffective
    D there is an immediate temporal connection between the impact of the exceptional stressor and the onset of symptoms
    E substance misuse commonly occurs

29.10   The main features of Ganser syndrome include:

    A vorbeigehen
    B full recollection after the event
    C hypochondriasis
    D pseudohallucinations
    E Gedankenlautwerden

Questions

30.1   The following are more common in women than in men:

   A   senile dementia
   B   completed suicide
   C   bulimia nervosa
   D   dysthymia
   E   alcoholism

30.2   In women there is an increase in the following during the premenstrual period:

   A   parasuicidal acts
   B   psychiatric hospital admissions
   C   shoplifting
   D   academic performance
   E   accidents

30.3   The prevalence of premenstrual symptoms is higher in those women:

   A   who have a monozygotic twin with premenstrual syndrome
   B   whose mothers have also suffered from premenstrual syndrome
   C   with type B behaviour compared with those with type A behaviour
   D   aged under 25 years
   E   who are nulliparous

30.4   Factors associated with miscarriage include:

   A   a severe life event in the preceding three months
   B   a major social difficulty
   C   increased social contacts
   D   fetal chromosomal abnormalities
   E   childhood maternal separation

30.5   Postnatal blues:

   A   is commonest between one and two weeks after childbirth
   B   usually lasts for one to two days
   C   occurs in up to 25% of women after childbirth
   D   is associated with poor social adjustment
   E   is associated with life events

30.6   The following statements concerning postnatal depression are correct:

    A it occurs in 25–35% of women after childbirth
    B it usually occurs within three months of childbirth
    C there is an increased risk of its development in women who are emotionally unstable in the first week after childbirth
    D there is an increased risk of its development in women who are nulliparous
    E genetic factors are important in its aetiology

30.7   The following are more frequent in the children of mothers suffering postnatal depression:

    A increased initial sociability
    B insecure attachment
    C behaviour problems
    D increased affective sharing
    E mild cognitive abnormalities

30.8   The following statements concerning puerperal psychosis are correct:

    A its onset is commonest within the first two days after childbirth
    B the organic psychotic type is commonest
    C after one episode of puerperal psychosis the risk of a further episode following a subsequent pregnancy is around 40–50%
    D it is preferable to treat the patient at home where she can look after her baby
    E lithium may be safely used in the treatment of lactating mothers

31 Sexual Disorders

Questions

31.1 The following statements concerning the ICD-10 disorder 'Lack of sexual enjoyment' are correct:

A it is more common in women than in men
B orgasm is not experienced
C it includes the diagnosis 'anhedonia (sexual)'
D it includes the diagnosis 'failure of genital response'
E in affected men penile erection occurs normally

31.2 Erectile dysfunction may be caused by:

A phenothiazines
B diabetes mellitus
C Peyronie's disease
D plumbism
E mumps

31.3 Premature ejaculation:

A is worsened by anxiety
B is treatable by the pause (stop–start) technique
C may respond to the squeeze technique
D is a side-effect of treatment with fluoxetine
E a common sign of sexual deviation

31.4 The following statements concerning orgasmic dysfunction in women are correct:

A it is more common than in men
B it may result from opiate use
C it is a side-effect of tricyclic antidepressants
D it is often associated with a fear of pregnancy and/or sexually transmitted diseases
E it is treatable by masturbatory training

31.5 The ICD-10 disorder 'non-organic vaginismus':

A is usually a secondary reaction
B is treatable with the squeeze technique
C is the primary presentation in around one in 10 women presenting to a sexual disorders clinic
D may respond to finger insertion
E results from spasm of the muscles that surround the vagina

31.6   The following statements concerning dual-role transvestism are correct:

   A it is a variant of fetishism
   B sexual excitement accompanies cross-dressing
   C there is a strong desire for membership of the opposite sex
   D it is often treated with surgical reassignment
   E patients are commonly hermaphrodites

31.7   The following statements concerning gender identity disorder of childhood in men
        are true:

   A it is first manifest before the onset of puberty in 50–80% of cases in clinical
          samples
   B it is commonly associated with a repudiation of one's own male anatomical
          structures
   C during adolescence, cross-dressing leads to sexual excitement
   D female dolls are often a favourite toy
   E patients commonly show a homosexual orientation during and after adolescence

31.8   The following statements concerning exhibitionism are true:

   A it occurs roughly equally in men and women
   B exposure is usually to strangers of the opposite sex
   C exposure by men is commonly followed by masturbation
   D the urges are usually ego-alien
   E the excitement experienced by the perpetrator is often heightened if the victim
          appears shocked, frightened or impressed

31.9   Recognized disorders of sexual preference include:

   A television oculophilia
   B frotteurism
   C sexual aversion
   D anoxophilia
   E telephone scatalogia

31.10   The following types of rapists are recognized:

   A situational
   B depressive
   C withdrawn
   D sociopathic
   E sexually inadequate

32 SLEEP DISORDERS

Questions

32.1 Compared with narcolepsy, in non-organic hypersomnia it is more likely that:

A cataplexy is present
B sleep paralysis is present
C hypnagogic hallucinations are present
D sleep attacks are irresistible
E nocturnal sleep is uninterrupted

32.2 Compared with narcolepsy, daytime sleep attacks in hypersomnia are more likely to be:

A fewer per day
B of shorter duration
C of gradual onset
D in unusual places
E accompanied by a typically sleep-onset REM EEG pattern

32.3 Parasomnias include:

A insomnia
B disorder of the sleep–wake schedule
C headbanging
D non-organic hypersomnia
E bruxism

32.4 Somnambulism usually:

A occurs during the second half of nocturnal sleep
B lasts more than one hour
C is followed by recall of what has transpired
D occurs during stages 1 and 2 of sleep
E occurs in adults

32.5 Sleep terrors usually:

A arise out of stages 3 and 4 of sleep
B occur during the first third of nocturnal sleep
C are associated with high levels of autonomic discharge
D last at least 20 minutes
E are associated with intense vocalization

32.6   Nightmares usually:

    A arise out of stages 3 and 4 of sleep
    B occur during the first third of nocturnal sleep
    C are associated with autonomic discharge
    D are associated with appreciable body motility
    E are associated with intense vocalization

32.7   The following statements concerning sleep paralysis are correct:

    A its onset is usually gradual
    B its onset is usually during awakening
    C the paralysis is usually flaccid
    D episodes usually last less than one minute
    E it may be accompanied by hallucinatory voices

32.8   The Kleine–Levin syndrome is characteristically associated with:

    A anorexia
    B urinary incontinence
    C hyposexuality
    D marked irritability
    E increased prolactin levels

33 PERSONALITY DISORDERS

Questions

33.1 Henderson's classification of psychopathic states included the following subtypes:

A creative psychopaths
B antisocial
C eccentric
D aggressive
E untruthful

33.2 The following people are correctly paired with their contribution to the development of the concept of personality disorder:

A Pritchard–manie sans délire
B Kraeplin–moral insanity
C Schneider–psychopathic personalities
D Tyrer–PAS
E Pinel–psychopathic personality

33.3 The following people are correctly paired with their contribution to the understanding of personality:

A Kelly–personal construct theory
B Roger–repertory grid
C Cattell–trait theory
D Eysenck–MMPI
E Bannister–self-theory

33.4 Criteria for making an ICD-10 diagnosis of schizoid personality disorder include:

A few, if any, activities provide pleasure
B emotional coldness
C tendency to bear grudges persistently
D limited capacity to express either warm, tender feelings or anger towards others
E apparent indifference to either praise or criticism

33.5 Criteria for making an ICD-10 diagnosis of histrionic personality disorder include:

A self-dramatization, theatricality, exaggerated expression of emotions
B callous unconcern for the feelings of others
C shallow and labile affectivity
D suggestibility
E gross and persistent attitude of irresponsibility and disregard for social norms, rules and obligations

33.6   Criteria for making an ICD-10 diagnosis of paranoid personality disorder include:

    A   insensitivity to social norms and conventions
    B   lack of desire for close friends or confiding relationships
    C   suspicious, misconstrues actions as hostile
    D   over-concern with physical attractiveness
    E   combative, tenacious sense of personal rights

33.7   Criteria for making an ICD-10 diagnosis of dissocial personality disorder include:

    A   suspicions regarding fidelity of partner
    B   excessive self-importance
    C   callous unconcern for feelings of others
    D   gross and persistent irresponsibility and disregard for social norms, rules and
        obligations
    E   incapacity to maintain enduring relationships

33.8   Criteria for making an ICD-10 diagnosis of anankastic personality disorder include:

    A   feelings of excessive doubt and caution
    B   marked proneness to blame others
    C   perfectionism interferes with task completion
    D   inappropriate seductiveness in appearance or behaviour
    E   rigid and stubborn

33.9   Criteria for making an ICD-10 diagnosis of anxious personality disorder include:

    A   persistent, pervasive tension and apprehension
    B   believe they are socially inept, unappealing or inferior to others
    C   preoccupation with being criticized or rejected in social situations
    D   continual seeking for excitement
    E   incapacity to experience guilt and to profit from experience

33.10   Criteria for making an ICD-10 diagnosis of dependent personality disorder include:

    A   intrusion of unwelcome, insistent thoughts or impulses
    B   encouraging or allowing others to make most of one's important life decisions
    C   preoccupation with conspiratorial explanations of events
    D   very low tolerance of frustration and a low threshold for discharge of aggression
    E   preoccupation with details, rules, lists, order, organization or schedule

33.11   The following statements concerning antisocial personality disorder are correct:

      A there is a higher prevalence in inner cities than in rural areas

      B the highest lifetime prevalence is in those aged 18–24 years

      C spontaneous remission may occurr in middle age

      D patients are more likely to be married than unmarried

      E there is a significant correlation with drug and alcohol dependence

Questions

34.1 Behavioural and emotional problems in preschool children:

A are more common in girls
B have a prevalence of up to 5%
C are strongly associated with maternal depression
D are strongly associated with poor parental marriage
E are strongly associated with delayed development of language

34.2 The Isle of Wight study of 10- and 11-year-olds by Rutter and his colleagues found that the:

A overall point prevalence of child psychiatric disorder was between 10% and 15%
B prevalence of child psychiatric disorder was greater in boys than in girls
C point prevalence of conduct disorder was around 4%
D point prevalence of emotional disorder was around 5%
E overall point prevalence of child psychiatric disorder was twice that found in a similar study of children in inner London

34.3 The ICD-10 classification 'Emotional disorders with onset specific to childhood' includes:

A depressive conduct disorder
B separation anxiety disorder of childhood
C elective mutism
D phobic anxiety of childhood
E social anxiety disorder of childhood

34.4 The ICD-10 classification 'Other behavioural and emotional disorders with onset usually occurring in childhood and adolescence' includes:

A hyperkinetic conduct disorder
B disinhibited attachment disorder of childhood
C Gilles de la Tourette syndrome
D pica of infancy and childhood
E non-organic encopresis

34.5   The following statements concerning school refusal are correct:

A it is more common in boys than in girls
B an incidence peak occurs at 5 years of age
C an incidence peak occurs at 13 years of age
D in adolescence it may be a symptom of depressive disorder
E it may be treated using the Kennedy approach

34.6   Truancy differs from school refusal in that it is:

A ego-dystonic
B rarely accompanied by other antisocial symptoms
C more likely to be associated with a family history of antisocial behaviour
D more likely to be associated with poor academic school performance
E more likely to be associated with increased family size

34.7   The following statements concerning hyperkinetic disorder are correct:

A it is more common in boys
B there is an increased incidence with increased social adversity
C the point prevalence is around 20–25%
D impaired attention is a cardinal feature
E central nervous system stimulants are commonly used in its treatment

34.8   The following statements concerning elective mutism are correct:

A it is more common in boys
B its prevalence is less than 1 per 1000 children
C it usually manifests in early childhood
D in general, it has a poor long-term prognosis
E it is commonly associated with social anxiety

34.9   The following statements concerning Tourette's syndrome are correct:

A it is more common in boys
B the lifetime prevalence is less than 0.1%
C the average age of onset is 15 years
D first-degree relatives often have multiple tics
E the majority present initially with vocal tics

34.10   The following statements concerning non-organic encopresis are correct:

    A the passage of faeces is not voluntary
    B it is more common in boys
    C it was found to have a prevalence of greater than 1% in boys aged 12 years in the Isle of Wight study
    D in the continuous encopresis subtype, bowel control has never been achieved
    E it has a poor prognosis

35 LEARNING DISABILITY

Questions

35.1   In ICD-10, aspects of the diagnosis of moderate mental retardation include:

A the IQ range is 30–49
B subjects have little or no self-care
C it is often associated with epilepsy, neurological and other disability
D independent living is rarely achieved
E any behavioural, social and emotional difficulties are similar to the 'normal'

35.2   The ICD-10 category 'Specific developmental disorders of speech and language' includes:

A expressive language disorder
B specific reading disorder
C specific spelling disorder
D mixed specific developmental disorders
E acquired aphasia with epilepsy

35.3   The ICD-10 category 'Pervasive developmental disorders' includes:

A Tourette's syndrome
B AD/HD
C Rett's syndrome
D schizophrenia of childhood onset
E Asperger's syndrome

35.4   The following statements concerning childhood autism are correct:

A the sex ratio is equal
B poor or absent social interaction is a characteristic feature
C poor eye contact is a characteristic feature
D it is commonly associated with echolalia
E it is commonly associated with socioemotional reciprocity

35.5   The following statements concerning Down's syndrome are correct:

A bradycephaly is not a feature
B curvature of the middle finger commonly occurs
C the IQ is less than 35 in around 90% of cases
D hypotonia is a feature
E a high arched palate is a feature

35.6   Clinical features of fragile X syndrome include:

   A prognathism
   B small forehead
   C hard rough skin
   D high arched palate
   E macro-orchidism post-pubertally

36 EATING DISORDERS

Questions

36.1 An ICD-10 diagnosis of anorexia nervosa requires the presence of:

A amenorrhoea in women
B hypogonadism in men
C Quetelet's body mass index of less than 16 kg m^{-2}
D body-image distortion
E self-imposed low weight threshold

36.2 Physical signs and complications commonly seen in anorexia nervosa include:

A peripheral oedema
B dehydration
C mitral valve prolapse
D raised blood pressure
E diarrhoea

36.3 Blood biochemical abnormalities that commonly occur in anorexia nervosa include:

A hyperglycaemia
B hypercholesterolaemia
C hyperkalaemia
D metabolic acidosis
E hypercarotaemia

36.4 Haematological abnormalities commonly seen in anorexia nervosa include:

A macrocytosis
B reduced MCH
C reduced haemoglobin level
D leucopenia
E a relative lymphocytosis

36.5 The following statements concerning anorexia nervosa are correct:

A the female to male ratio is around 10:1
B the peak incidence occurs between 15 and 19 years of age
C the prevalence is 10–20 per 1000 women
D there is a reduced prevalence in higher socioeconomic classes
E there is an increased prevalence in ballet and modelling schools

36.6   Physical signs commonly occurring in bulimia nervosa that may result from vomiting include:

A   Russell's sign
B   parotid gland enlargement
C   oedema
D   conjunctival haemorrhages
E   toothache

36.7   The following statements concerning bulimia nervosa are correct:

A   the female to male ratio is around 10:1
B   the average age of onset is less than that for anorexia nervosa
C   the prevalence in adolescence and young adult women is around 10–30 per 1000
D   the lifetime prevalence is around 1% for women
E   the concordance rate for monozygotic twins is not significantly different to that for dizygotic twins

37 CROSS-CULTURAL PSYCHIATRY

Questions

37.1   The International Pilot Study of Schizophrenia:

A   was conducted by the American Psychiatric Association
B   was conducted in the 1980s
C   included the UK as a centre studied
D   included Sweden as a centre studied
E   showed that the incidence of schizophrenia, narrowly defined according to Schneider's first-rank symptoms, was approximately equal across the countries studied

37.2   Amok:

A   occurs mainly in Malays
B   is more common in women
C   is commonly followed by amnesia for the event
D   has an initial period of withdrawal
E   attacks typically last several hours

37.3   The following statements concerning koro are correct:

A   it occurs in South-East Asia and China
B   it is more common in women
C   it usually includes a fear of impending death
D   it usually includes a period of homicidal aggression
E   the attack usually comes to an end after the person has killed themselves or been killed by others

37.4   The following statements concerning dhat are correct:

A   it commonly occurs in Malaya
B   it is more common in women
C   automatic obedience is a feature
D   the subject usually has a fear of impending death
E   lack of literacy is an important predisposing factor

37.5   The following statements concerning windigo are correct:

A   it occurs mainly in Eskimos
B   it may be ascribed to schizophrenia
C   it may be ascribed to depression
D   the subject typically tears off their clothing and screams and runs wildly
E   the subject often presents with sexual dysfunction

37.6   The following statements concerning latah are correct:

    A it occurs in the Far East and North Africa
    B it is more common in women
    C it is an hysterical state
    D coprolalia is often a feature
    E echopraxia is often a feature

37.7   The following statements concerning brain fag syndrome are correct:

    A it is seen particularly in North American Indians
    B it usually begins following a sudden frightening experience
    C ocular symptoms are a common feature
    D aching, burning or crawling sensations in the head commonly occur
    E it responds well to psychological interpretation

38 OLD AGE PSYCHIATRY

Questions

38.1   In the elderly, compared with younger adults, characteristic changes that may affect pharmacokinetics include:

A   an increase in the proportion of body mass that is composed of water
B   a decrease in the proportion of body mass that is composed of muscle
C   a decrease in gastric pH
D   reduced hepatic biotransformation
E   reduced glomerular filtration rate

38.2   Compared with younger adults, features of tricyclic antidepressant treatment in the elderly include:

A   an increased plasma half-life
B   an increased steady-state level
C   a reduced volume of distribution
D   a reduced risk of postural hypotension
E   reduced sensitivity to antimuscarinic side-effects

38.3   Psychometric tests that are of particular use in assessing elderly patients include the:

A   Kew Cognitive Map
B   WISC-R
C   CAPE
D   Kendrick Battery
E   WPPSI

38.4   Features that often develop in the early and intermediate stages of Alzheimer's disease include:

A   epilepsy
B   echolalia
C   catastrophic reactions
D   the mirror sign
E   emotional lability

38.5   Leukoaraiosis:

   A   is a clinical diagnosis
   B   is commoner in Alzheimer's disease than in multi-infarct dementia
   C   is significantly associated with limb weakness
   D   is significantly associated with lower blood pressure
   E   commonly occurs in the temporoparietal cortex

38.6   Variant forms of Creutzfeldt–Jakob disease include:

   A   Lewy body form
   B   heidenhain form
   C   thalamic form
   D   ataxic form
   E   cortical form

38.7   The following statements concerning general paralysis of the insane are correct:

   A   it usually develops up to five years after the primary infection
   B   the onset is usually gradual
   C   most patients have grandiose delusions
   D   depression is a dominant symptom
   E   slurred speech is common

39 FORENSIC PSYCHIATRY

Questions

39.1   Juvenile delinquency:

    A refers to reduced intelligence in juveniles
    B refers to those aged 13–17 years
    C is associated with unsatisfactory child rearing
    D is associated with being an only child
    E is associated with parental criminality

39.2   The following statements concerning the epidemiology of offending in the UK are correct:

    A the peak age of offending is higher in women than in men
    B men are more commonly convicted than are women
    C around one-half of all indictable crimes are committed by people under the age of 21 years
    D after the age of 30 years, the rate of offending gradually continues to decrease in women
    E by the age of 30 years, around 30% of men have been convicted of an indictable offence

39.3   In England and Wales, criminal responsibility:

    A starts earlier than in Scotland
    B starts at the age of 12 years
    C is partial up to the age of 13 years
    D that is partial is referred to as Dolci Incapax
    E refers to the fact that after the age that a person becomes fully criminally responsible, they are always legally responsible for their actions

39.4   In England and Wales, the outcome of sentencing of mentally abnormal offenders can include:

    A imprisonment
    B a conditional discharge
    C a probation order with a condition of psychiatric treatment
    D dentention under the Mental Health Act
    E the imposition of a fine

39.5   A mentally disordered offender may be considered to be unfit to plead as a result of:

    A the fact that they were suffering from schizophrenia at the time of the offence
    B being unable to challenge a juror
    C being unable to give oral evidence in court
    D being unable to examine a witness in court
    E being unable to understand and follow the evidence of court procedure

39.6   Types of unlawful homicide include:

    A the killing of another as a result of a pure accident
    B infanticide
    C murder
    D killing on behalf of the state
    E manslaughter

39.7   The following statements concerning kleptomania are correct:

    A it is classified in the category 'other disorders of adult personality and behaviour' in ICD-10
    B it is commonly found in arrested shoplifters
    C the average age of onset is around 14 years
    D the diagnosis is usually made in people in their early 20s
    E the offences are usually carried out with long-term planning and assistance

39.8   A marriage may be annulled if:

    A the partner had a mental disorder at the time of the marriage so as not to appreciate the nature of the contract
    B one partner did not disclose that they suffered from epilepsy before the marriage
    C the husband battered his wife
    D there was non-consummation
    E one partner did not disclose that they suffered from a communicable venereal disease before the marriage

PART TWO

Answers

1 BASIC PSYCHOLOGY

Answers

1.1

A True

According to this theory, internal discomfort occurs when two or more cognitions are held but are inconsistent with each other.

B False

When cognitive dissonance occurs, the individual feels uncomfortable, may experience increased arousal and is motivated to achieve cognitive consistency.

C False

This theory was first formulated by Festinger.

D False

While cognitive dissonance includes the situation in which the subject has cognitions that are not consistent with behavioural tendencies, the term used to describe the situation when attitude and behaviour are inconsistent is attitude-discrepant behaviour.

E True

The subject is motivated to achieve cognitive consistency, and this may occur through changes in cognition or behaviour.

References/Further Reading

Revision Notes in Psychiatry, pp. 9 and 13.
Sciences Basic to Psychiatry, 1st edn, pp. 286–7.

1.2

A True

By reinforcing successively closer approximations, a desired behaviour can be achieved. This process, known as shaping, finds application clinically in the management of behavioural disturbances in people with learning difficulties.

B False

Classical conditioning and operant conditioning are both forms of associative learning.

C False

Operant conditioning is based on work by Thorndike and, later, Skinner involving trial-and-error learning or behaviour in animals.

D False

Negative reinforcement is not the same as punishment. In the context of operant conditioning, negative reinforcement refers to the reinforcement of a response through the removal of a negative reinforcer (a negative reinforcer is an aversive stimulus, the removal of which increases the probability of occurrence of the operant behaviour). Punishment, on the other hand, is the situation that occurs if an aversive stimulus is presented whenever a given behaviour occurs.

E True

In continuous reinforcement, reinforcement takes place following every condtioned response; it leads to the maximum response rate. In partial reinforcement with a fixed interval schedule, on the other hand, reinforcement only takes place after a fixed interval of time; such a schedule is poor at maintaining the conditioned response and the maximum response rate tends to occur only when the reinforcement is expected.

References/Further Reading

Revision Notes in Psychiatry, pp. 2–3.
Sciences Basic to Psychiatry, 1st edn, pp. 280–2.

1.3

A True

Habituation is an important component of the behavioural treatment of obsessive–compulsive disorder using exposure and response prevention.

B False

Imprinting refers to a process described by the ethologist Lorenz in, for example, geese, whereby the first nearby moving object encountered during a critical period soon after hatching is then persistently followed around. It is normally species specific.

C True

Reciprocal inhibition holds that relaxation inhibits anxiety so that the two are mutually exclusive. It can be used in treating conditions such as phobias associated with anticipatory anxiety.

D True

In shaping, successively closer approximations to the desired behaviour are reinforced in order to achieve the desired behaviour. It finds application clinically in the management of behavioural disturbances in people with learning difficulties.

E True

In chaining, the components of a more complex desired behaviour are first taught and then connected in order to teach the desired behaviour. It can be used in, for example, people with learning difficulties.

References/Further Reading

Revision Notes in Psychiatry, p. 3.
Sciences Basic to Psychiatry, 1st edn, pp. 275–6.

False

Escape conditioning is a variety of negative reinforcement in which the response learnt provides complete escape from the aversive stimulus.

B True

An optimal condition for vicarious learning (observational learning) is that the subject sees that the behaviour observed is being reinforced.

C False

Maximum likelihood estimation is an estimation procedure used in statistics.

D False

While learning may be defined as a change in behaviour resulting from prior experience, it does not include behavioural change caused by temporary conditions such as drug effects.

E True

An optimal condition for vicarious learning is perceived similarity – the subject must believe that he or she can emit the response necessary to obtain reinforcement.

References/Further Reading

Revision Notes in Psychiatry, pp. 1, 3 and 4.

1.5

A number of perceptual phenomena are described in Gestalt psychology:

- the whole perception is different from the sum of its parts
- law of simplicity
- law of closure
- law of continuity
- law of similarity
- law of proximity
- figure ground differentiation

A False

The law of effect is a concept in operant conditioning that was described by Thorndike. It holds that voluntary behaviour that is paired with subsequent reward is strengthened.

B True

The percept corresponds to the simplest stimulation interpretation.

C True

Adjacent items are grouped together.

D True

Patterns are perceived as figures differentiated from their background with contours and boundaries, thus simulating objects.

E False

Fechner's law holds that sensory perception is a logarithmic function of stimulus intensity.

References/Further Reading

Revision Notes in Psychiatry, pp. 2 and 4.

1.6

A False

Depth perception usually develops by around 2 months of age.

B True

A three-dimensional visual perception is formed from two-dimensional retinal images as a result of multiple cues, such as binocular vision and convergence, relative size and brightness, motion parallax, object interposition and linear perspective.

C True

Depth perception may be demonstrated in infants after the age of 2 months by placing them on a visual cliff consisting of a thick sheet of glass overlying two similarly patterned surfaces positioned at different heights, one directly under the glass and the other a relatively large drop below. An infant with intact depth perception placed on a board between the two regions will not cross onto that part of the glass surface that covers the deeper region.

D True

There is disturbance of perception, particularly depth perception and perceptual constancy.

E True

There is disturbance of perception, particularly depth perception and perceptual constancy.

References/Further Reading

Revision Notes in Psychiatry, p. 5.

1.7

A True

Figure ground discrimination is believed to be innate.

B False

This is not an aspect of visual perception. A haptic memory refers to the sensory memory for information from touch.

C True

Visual fixating is believed to be innate.

D False

Size constancy is believed to be learnt.

E False

Shape discrimination is believed to be learnt.

References/Further Reading

Revision Notes in Psychiatry, pp. 5 and 7.

1.8

Attention is an intensive process in which information selection takes place. Types include:

- selective/focused attention
- divided attention
- sustained attention
- controlled attention
- automatic
- Stroop effect.

A False

This is a process involved primarily with memory rather than attention, in which the probability of correctly recalling an item of information is increased if it is one of the most recent items to be encountered.

B False

This process is involved primarily with memory rather than attention, and refers to the fading of memory with time.

C True

The automatic process is so ingrained that it interferes with controlled processing.

D True

Dual-task interference refers to loss of performance occurring during divided attention.

E False

Chunking is a process involved primarily with memory rather than attention. It serves to increase the amount of information stored in short-term memory by allowing one entry to cover several items.

References/Further Reading

Revision Notes in Psychiatry, pp. 6, 7 and 8.

1.9

Long-term memory or secondary memory stores information more or less permanently and theoretically may have unlimited capacity, although there may be limitations on retrieval.

A False

This is short-term memory.

B False

Echoic memory is the sensory memory for auditory information.

C False

Sensory memory is a very short-lived trace of the sensory input.

D True

This is long-term memory for events. It provides a continually changing and updated record of autobiographical material.

E False

This is short-term memory.

References/Further Reading

Revision Notes in Psychiatry, pp. 6–7.

1.10

Theories based on instincts were replaced by a drive reduction theory in which the motivation of behaviour is to reduce the level of arousal associated with a basic drive (biological drive, e.g. hunger and thirst) in order to maintain homeostatic control of the internal somatic environment.

A True

Secondary drives may result from generalization.

B True

Secondary drives may result from conditioning.

C False

Thirst is a primary biological drive.

D True

Anxiety is a secondary drive.

E False

The concept of secondary drives was developed primarily by Mowrer. Hull developed a theory in which primary biological drives are activated by needs that arise from homeostatic imbalance acting via brain receptors.

References/Further Reading

Revision Notes in Psychiatry, p. 8.

1.11

Whereas extrinsic theories require reduction of drive externally, intrinsic theories propose that the activity engaged in has its own intrinsic reward. Intrinsic motivation theories include:

- optimal arousal
- cognitive dissonance
- attitude-discrepant behaviour
- need for achievement (nAch).

A True

The subject attains an optimal level of arousal to achieve optimal performance. In general a moderate level of arousal leads to an optimum degree of alertness and interest, and therefore to a comparatively high efficiency of performance, while high and low arousal lead to reduced performance.

B False

This relates to extrinsic motivation. In the drive reduction theory the motivation of behaviour is to reduce the level of arousal associated with a basic drive in order to maintain homeostatic control of the internal somatic environment.

C True

This explains pleasure resulting from mastery.

D True

The individual is motivated to achieve cognitive consistency and may change one or more of the cognitions.

E True

Alteration of attitude helps bring about cognitive consistency.

References/Further Reading

Revision Notes in Psychiatry, pp. 8–9.

1.12

A True

James was a Harvard psychologist who helped formulate the theory now known as the James–Lange theory, according to which the experience of emotion is secondary to the somatic responses to the perception of given emotionally important events. For example, if an arachnophobe becomes aroused, experiences increased activity of the sympathetic nervous system and runs away after seeing a spider, the feelings of anxiety and fear are the result of the increased sympathetic activity and running away, and not primarily because of the emotion-evoking stimulus.

B True

Independently of James (see **A** above), the Danish physiologist Lange also helped formulate the theory now known as the James–Lange theory.

C True

Cannon criticized the James–Lange theory. It was argued that similar physiological changes can accompany different emotions. Also, pharmacologically induced simulation of such physiological changes is usually not accompanied by these emotions. The experience of emotions can be shown to be independent of somatic responses, sometimes occurring before the somatic responses. He helped formulate the theory now known as the Cannon–Bard theory (see **D** below).

D True

Bard helped formulate the theory now known as the Cannon–Bard theory. This holds that following the perception of an emotionally important event both the somatic responses and the experience of emotion occur together. In neurophysiological terms, the perceived stimulus undergoes thalamic processing, and signals are then relayed to both the cerebral cortex, leading to the experience of emotion, and other parts of the body, such as the autonomic nervous system, leading to somatic responses.

E True

Schachter's cognitive labelling theory holds that the conscious experience of an emotion is a function of the stimulus, of somatic or physiological responses, and of cognitive factors such as the cognitive appraisal of the situation and input from long-term memory. The influence of cognitive factors on the conscious experience of emotion was demonstrated in an experiment by Schachter and Singer in which subjects were injected with adrenaline. Their cognitive appraisal of the current situation, based on observation of others, influenced the conscious experience of emotion. Thus cognitive cues were important in their interpretation of arousal.

References/Further Reading

Revision Notes in Psychiatry, pp. 9–10.

1.13

A False

Love is a secondary emotion derived from the primary emotions of joy and acceptance.

B True

Plutchik classified emotions into the following eight primary ones: disgust, anger, anticipation, joy, acceptance, fear, surprise and sadness.

C False

Submission is a secondary emotion derived from the primary emotions of acceptance and fear.

D True

See **A** and **C** above.

E True

See **B** above.

References/Further Reading

Revision Notes in Psychiatry, p. 9.

1.14

Although the following coping mechanisms, used to cope with stress, are conscious, they also relate to unconscious defence mechanisms (given in parentheses):

- concentration only on the current task (denial)
- empathy (projection)
- logical analysis (rationalization)
- objectivity (isolation)
- playfulness (regression)
- substitution of other thoughts for disturbing ones (reaction formation)
- suppression of inappropriate feelings (repression).

A False

The conscious coping mechanism of empathy relates to the unconscious defence mechanism of projection.

B True

C True

D False

The conscious coping mechanism of objectivity relates to the unconscious defence mechanism of isolation.

E True

References/Further Reading

Revision Notes in Psychiatry, p. 11.

Answers

2.1

A True

Attitudes may be measured with a Likert scale (in which the intervals between each of the scores is equal).

B True

Beliefs constitute one of the main components of attitudes.

C True

Of the three main components of attitudes (see also **B** and **E**), the affective components are the most resistant to change.

D True

Attitudes are mutually consistent and internally consistent.

E True

Attitudes are based on a tendency to behave in an observable way.

References/Further Reading

Revision Notes in Psychiatry, p. 12.

2.2

A True

Message repetition can be a persuasive influence leading to attitude change.

B False

Explicit messages are more persuasive for the less intelligent and implicit messages for the more intelligent recipient.

C True

Being an opinion leader is a characteristic of persuasive communicators.

D True

Interactive personal discussions are more persuasive than mass media communication.

E False

One-sided communications are more persuasive for those who are less intelligent while two-sided presentations are more effective with intelligent recipients.

References/Further Reading

Revision Notes in Psychiatry, p. 13.

2.3

A False

The balance theory holds that each individual attempts to organize his or her attitudes, perceptions, and beliefs so that they are in harmony or balance with each other.

B True

According to this theory, the preferred relationships are those in which each feels that the cost–benefit ratio of the relationship for each person is approximately equal.

C False

This theory deals with the rules people use to infer the causes of observed behaviour.

D True

According to this theory, reciprocal reinforcement of attractions occurs with rewards in both directions. Conversely, punishments diminish the probability of interpersonal attraction.

E True

This relates to the interpersonal space–body buffer zone.

References/Further Reading

Revision Notes in Psychiatry, pp. 13 and 14.

2.4

A True

In this type, the person is charismatic and liked by others.

B True

In this type, the person has the power to punish.

C False

Normative social influence refers to situations in which an individual publicly conforms to the consensual opinion and behaviour of the group but has a different view in his or her own mind. The individual conforms to the group under social pressure to avoid social rejection.

D True

In this type, the person has power derived from their role.

E True

In this type, the person has power derived from skill, knowledge and experience.

References/Further Reading

Revision Notes in Psychiatry, p. 15.

2.5

A False

This is the inference that the cause of a behaviour is external to the person. It is also known as external attribution.

B True

This is one of the conditions that Cook showed as needing to be satisfied in order to reduce prejudice.

C False

On the contrary, the potential for personal acquaintance is more likely to reduce prejudice. With respect to animal behaviour, ethological studies have shown that maintaining a distance may inhibit aggression.

D True

This is one of the conditions that Cook showed as needing to be satisfied in order to reduce prejudice.

E True

This is one of the conditions that Cook showed as needing to be satisfied in order to reduce prejudice.

References/Further Reading

Revision Notes in Psychiatry, pp. 14 and 16.

Answers

3.1

Explicit memory requires a deliberate act of recollection and can be reported verbally. It includes declarative memory and episodic memory, which are probably stored separately, as it is possible to lose one type of memory while retaining the other. Declarative memory involves knowledge of facts, whereas episodic memory involves memory of autobiographical events. Explicit memory involves the medial temporal lobes, particularly the hippocampus, entorhinal cortex, subiculum and parahippocampal cortex. Damage to these structures results in an inability to store new memory. Memory probably passes from medial temporal lobe structures after a few weeks or months to longer term storage in the cortex.

A False

Explicit memory is a type of long-term memory; the latter can be considered to be made up of explicit memory and implicit memory.

B False

Explicit memory requires a deliberate act of recollection.

C True

D True

E True

References/Further Reading

Revision Notes in Psychiatry, p. 18.

3.2

Implicit memory is recalled automatically without effort and is learnt slowly through repetition. It is not readily amenable to verbal reporting.

A True

B True

C False

Implicit memory comprises procedural knowledge, i.e. knowing how. (It is declarative memory that involves knowledge of facts; declarative memory is a type of explicit memory.)

D True

Its storage requires functioning of the cerebellum, amygdala and specific sensory and motor systems used in the learned task. (For example, the basal ganglia are involved in learning motor skills.)

E True

Both classical and operant learning involve implicit memory.

References/Further Reading

Revision Notes in Psychiatry, p. 18.

3.3

> 'Geschwind ... provided a model [of language functioning] based upon the learning and arousal of associative links. He pointed out that the distinctive element in human language, which is not present in animal communication, derives from man's ability to form higher-order associations between one sensory stimulus and another...The impressive advance in the human brain lies in the expansion of the zone in the region of the angular gyrus at the junction of the temporal, parietal and occipital lobes, which is an area strategically situated with respect to the association cortices for hearing, touch and vision.'
>
> Lishman, W.A. (1998) *Organic Psychiatry: The Psychological Consequences of Cerebral Disorder*, 3rd edn. Oxford: Blackwell Science.

A False

The left cerebral hemisphere is dominant in around 60% of left-handers, while in 99% of right-handers the left cerebral hemisphere is dominant.

B False

In early life there is plasticity for cerebral dominance for language before the functions are established.

C True

The angular gyrus (BA 39) has abundant connections with the somatosensory, visual and auditory association cortices. An inability to read is a characteristic feature of lesions of the angular gyrus; the pathway for understanding written language, i.e. reading, is as follows:

written word → visual cortex → visual association cortex → angular gyrus → Wernicke's area → read and comprehend.

D True

As in **C** above, an inability to write is a characteristic feature of lesions of the angular gyrus; the pathway for writing is as follows:

thought/cognition → Wernicke's area → angular gyrus → motor areas → write.

E False

The auditory association cortex is found in the temporal lobe.

References/Further Reading

Organic Psychiatry, 3rd edn, pp. 43–5.
Revision Notes in Psychiatry, pp. 18–19.

3.4

Damage to Wernicke's area disrupts ability to comprehend language, either written or spoken. In addition to loss of comprehension, the person also is unaware that their dysphasic speech is difficult for others to follow. The content of speech is abnormal. Words used have lost their meaning; empty words (e.g. 'thing', 'it') and paraphrasias are used liberally.

A False

Speech is normal in intonation because Broca's area is intact.

B False

Speech is normal in rhythm because Broca's area is intact.

C False

Damage to Wernicke's area results in a fluent receptive dysphasia. (Expressive dysphasia can result from damage to Broca's area.)

D True

As mentioned in Answer 3.3, the pathway for understanding written language, i.e. reading, is as follows:

written word → visual cortex → visual association cortex → angular gyrus → Wernicke's area → read and comprehend.

E True

References/Further Reading

Revision Notes in Psychiatry, pp. 19.

3.5

Damage to the arcuate fasciculus results in a conduction dysphasia in which the person cannot repeat what is said to them. Their comprehension and verbal fluency remain intact.

A True

B False

The pathway for understanding spoken language is as follows:

spoken word → auditory cortex → auditory association cortex → Wernicke's area → hear and comprehend speech.

C True

D True

E False

References/Further Reading

Revision Notes in Psychiatry, p. 19.

3.6

Perception relates to the means by which the brain makes representations of the external environment. So far as visual perception is concerned, the determination of shape, colour and spatial orientation takes place in the occipital lobes. Lesions at this level result in pseudoagnosia.

A True

B True

C False

Visuospatial elements are drawn together into complete percepts, in which objects are perceived as a whole, in the right (non-dominant) parietal lobe. However, meaning is not yet attributed to the objects at this level.

D True

E False

The attribution of meaning in visual perception is not a function solely of the occipital lobes. It is believed that parieto-occipital areas play an important part in this function, with meaning being accessed from the left (dominant) parietal lobe (which itself accesses meaning from semantic memory).

References/Further Reading

Revision Notes in Psychiatry, p. 20.

3.7

A False

In visual perception, visuospatial elements are drawn together into complete percepts, whereby objects are perceived as a whole, in the right (non-dominant) parietal lobe. Meaning is not yet attributed to the objects at this level. Lesions at this level result in apperceptive agnosia.

B True

In anosognosia there is a lack of awareness of disease, particularly of hemiplegia (most often following a right parietal lesion).

C False

In visual perception, associative agnosia may result from lesions (usually bilateral) at the level of the parieto-occipital areas. It sometimes also involves the posterior temporal lobes. However, it is not a characteristic feature of solely dominant temporal lobe lesions. Unlike apperceptive agnosics, who cannot copy objects or drawings, associative agnosics may be able to produce reasonable drawings of objects (that they cannot identify).

D False

Expressive dysphasia is not an agnosia. The term agnosia was introduced by Sigmund Freud. Lishman quotes the definition by Frederiks (1969) of agnosia being an impaired recognition of an object that is sensorially presented, while at the same time the impairment cannot be reduced to sensory defects, mental deterioration, disorders of consciousness and attention, or to a non-familiarity with the object.

E True

Achromatopsia is a form of colour agnosia in which there is a profound loss of colour sense extending even to an inability to imagine colours, the concept of colour itself being abolished. It is characteristically associated with damage in the occipital and subcalcarine portions of the lingual gyri bilaterally.

References/Further Reading

Frederiks, J.A.M. (1969) Disorders of the body schema. In: *Handbook of Clinical Neurology*, Vol. 4, Vinken, P.J. and Bruyn, G.W. (eds), Amsterdam: North-Holland Publishing Co.
Organic Psychiatry, 3rd edn, pp. 58–61.
Revision Notes in Psychiatry, p. 20.

3.8

Apraxia is an inability to perform purposive volitional acts, which does not result from paresis, incoordination, sensory loss or involuntary movements. The patient cannot at will set the movement in train or guide a series of consecutive movements in their correct spatial and temporal sequence, even though the same muscles can be used and analogous movements performed in other contexts.

A False

B False

C True

The patient is unable to carry out coordinated sequences of actions, such as taking a match from a box and striking it, or to perform the complex movements involved in using a pair of scissors or a comb, for example.

D True

E True

Constructional apraxia is closely associated with visuospatial agnosia.

References/Further Reading

Organic Psychiatry, 3rd edn, pp. 55–8.
Revision Notes in Psychiatry, p. 20.

3.9

A False

In simultanagnosia the patient is unable to recognize the overall meaning of a picture, whereas its individual details are understood.

B False

In agnosia for colours the patient is unable to name colours correctly, although colour sense is still present.

C True

Prosopagnosia is an inability to recognize faces. In advanced Alzheimer's disease a patient may misidentify their own mirrored reflection; this is known as the mirror sign.

D False

In astereognosia objects cannot be recognized by palpation. It is topographical disorientation that can be tested using a locomotor map-reading task in which the patient is asked to trace out a given route by foot.

E True

Agraphaesthesia or agraphognosia is tested by asking the patient to identify, with closed eyes, numbers or letters traced on his or her palm; this disorder is present if the patient is unable to identify such writing.

References/Further Reading

Revision Notes in Psychiatry, p. 20.

3.10

Gerstmann's syndrome is caused by dominant parietal lobe lesions and consists of:

*   dyscalculia
*   agraphia
*   finger agnosia
*   right–left disorientation.

A False

B True

This manifests as an inability to carry out instructions involving an appreciation of right and left. For example, the patient fails to point on command to objects on their right and their left, to indicate parts of their body on the right and the left, or to perform more complex instructions in which these directions form an integral part of the task.

C False

D True

This is shown by loss of ability to recognize, name, identify or select individual fingers, either on the patient's own body or on that of another person. While traditionally the patient is asked to point to named fingers or to name an individual finger, the presence of dysphasia may interfere with this test. An alternative test is one in which two fingers are simultaneously touched by the examiner and the patient is asked to state the number of fingers between those touched, first in practice sessions with open eyes, and then with closed eyes.

E True

This is an impairment of the capacity for calculation in patients who have previously shown no disorder of arithmetical faculties. Note that secondary dyscalculia may result from:

*   short-term memory defects
*   perseveration
*   concentration impairment.

References/Further Reading

Organic Psychiatry, 3rd edn, pp. 65–7.
Revision Notes in Psychiatry, p. 21.

3.11

Functions believed to be associated with the prefrontal cortex include:

- problem-solving
- perceptual judgement
- memory
- programming and planning of sequences of behaviour
- verbal regulation
- level of response emission
- adaptability of response pattern
- tertiary level of motor control.

(Note that there is a printing error in the first imprint of *Revision Notes in Psychiatry* – the frontal eye fields should have been printed as a separate heading; voluntary eye movements are a function of the frontal eye fields rather than of the prefrontal cortex.)

A False

This is believed to be a function of the orbital cortex.

B True

C True

D True

E False

This is believed to be a function of the orbital cortex.

References/Further Reading

Revision Notes in Psychiatry, p. 21.

3.12

Frontal lobe lesions cause:

- personality change
- perseveration
- utilization behaviour
- pallilalia
- impairment of attention, concentration and initiative
- aspontaneity, slowed psychomotor activity
- motor Jacksonian fits
- urinary incontinence
- contralateral spastic paresis
- aphasia
- primary motor aphasia
- motor agraphia
- anosmia
- ipsilateral optic atrophy.

A True

This is a perseverative error of speech that entails the reiterations of single words, usually with increasing frequency.

B False

Frontal lobe lesions may give rise to motor Jacksonian fits. The motor area is located in the precentral area of the frontal lobe, with the posterior region of the precentral area being the primary motor area, and the anterior region of the precentral area containing the premotor or secondary motor area. The somaesthetic areas, however, are located not in the frontal lobes but in the parietal lobes. The primary somaesthetic area is situated in the post-central gyrus while the secondary somaesthetic area lies in the superior lip of the posterior ramus of the lateral sulcus.

C True

Sphincteric incontinence may occur surprisingly early in view of the reasonable preservation of intellect that occurs.

D True

Frontal lobe lesions may cause distinctive changes of disposition and temperament, i.e. 'changes of personality'. These often include:

- disinhibition
- reduced social and ethical control
- sexual indiscretions
- poor judgement
- elevated mood
- lack of concern for the feelings of other people
- irritability.

E True

This may result from orbital lesions of the frontal lobe. Such lesions may also cause anosmia.

References/Further Reading

Organic Psychiatry, 3rd edn, p. 17.
Revision Notes in Psychiatry, p. 21.
Sciences Basic to Psychiatry, 2nd edn, pp. 13–16.

4 Psychological Assessment

Answers

4.1

A False

This is not a source of error in psychological assessment by interview. Scaling refers to the conversion of raw data into types of scores more readily understood, for example ranks, (per)centiles and standardized scores.

B False

The Hawthorne effect is a source of error in which the interviewer alters the situation by their presence.

C False

The response set is a source of error in which the person being interviewed has the tendency always to agree or to disagree with the questions asked.

D False

Extreme responding is a source of error in which the person being interviewed has the tendency of selecting extreme responses.

E False

The halo effect is a source of error in which the observer allows his or her preconception to influence the responses.

References/Further Reading

Revision Notes in Psychiatry, p. 22.

4.2

A True

Naturalistic observations involve the assessment of behaviour as it occurs with minimum interference by the observer. In time-sampling techniques the subject is observed during given time intervals at given times of the day or night. Naturalistic observations are used in the functional analysis of problem behaviours. This method is sometimes referred as ABC (for antecedents, behaviours, consequences).

B True

Defensiveness is a potential source of error in psychological assessment by interview in which the subject avoids giving too much self-related information.

C True

A norm is an average, common or standard performance under specified conditions. In norm-referencing, a test may be standardized to this norm. Criterion-referencing may also be used, a criterion being a set of scores against which a predictive test's success can be compared.

D True

Social desirability is a potential source of error in psychological assessment by interview in which the subject makes a choice of responses that they believe the interviewer desires. Social desirability may be reduced through the use of the forced-choice technique.

E True

Social desirability may be reduced through the inclusion of lie scales.

References/Further Reading

Revision Notes in Psychiatry, pp. 22–3.

4.3

A False

The WPPSI is the Weschler Preschool and Primary Scale of Intelligence. It is a modified version of the WAIS for use with children between the ages of 4 and 6 years and 6 months.

B False

The WISC-R is the Weschler Intelligence Scale for Children – Revised. It is a modified version of the WAIS for use with children between the ages of 5 and 15 years.

C False

The CHAID is the Chi-squared Automatic Interaction Detector statistical analysis software that performs segmentation modelling. It is included as part of the SPSS software package.

D True

The WAIS is the Wechsler Adult Intelligence Scale. It is a well-standardized test that gives both a verbal IQ (intelligence quotient) and a performance IQ.

E False

The concept of the mental age was devised by Binet as the average intellectual ability, as measured by the level of problem-solving and reasoning. The scale was devised such that the average range of scores corresponds to the chronological age. For children with a higher than average level of intelligence, the mental age is greater than the chronological age. Conversely, for children with a lower than average level of intelligence, the mental age is less than the chronological age. The Stanford–Binet test can be applied to each year, up to the age of 15 years.

References/Further Reading

Revision Notes in Psychiatry, pp. 23–4.

4.4

The WAIS (Wechsler Adult Intelligence Scale) or WAIS-R (Wechsler Adult Intelligence Scale – Revised) consists of 11 subtests. It is probably the test most often used for the assessment of intelligence in adults and is well standardized.

A False

There are six verbal subtests

- information
- comprehension
- arithmetic
- similarities
- digit span
- vocabulary.

B True

There are five performance subtests

- picture completion
- block design
- picture arrangement
- object assembly
- digit symbol.

C True

This subtest assesses the subject's ability to define correctly words of increasing complexity.

D True

This subtest assesses the subject's immediate attention span and sequencing ability.

E True

This subtest is a timed coding task in which numbers have to be associated with marks of various shapes. It assesses the subject's speed of learning and writing, attention and visual–verbal transformation.

References/Further Reading

Revision Notes in Psychiatry, p. 23.
Seminars in Psychology and the Social Sciences, pp. 115–116.

4.5

In projective tests of personality, the presented items have no one correct answer. The tests instead take the form of ambiguous stimuli, upon which the subject projects their personality. The reliability and validity of projective tests of personality have not been established.

A False

The California Psychological Inventory (CPI) is an objective test that allows the measurement of 18 traits that are part of normal personality, such as achievement, dominance, self-acceptance and sociability.

B True

In this test the subject is shown a series of ambiguous pictures and has to make up a story about each one.

C True

In this test, named after the Swiss psychiatrist Hermann Rorschach, the subject is shown a series of 10 cards displaying ambiguous complex inkblot-like pictures, some of which are in black and white and some of which are coloured. The subject relates what they see in each card, reporting in each case what the inkblot resembles. The responses may be scored according to the following categories:

- location – whether the response involves the entire inkblot or just some part thereof
- determinants – whether the subject responds to the shape of the inkblot, its colour or differences in texture and shading
- content – what the response represents.

D False

The Minnesota Multiphasic Personality Inventory (MMPI) is a standardized self-report personality inventory, consisting of around 550 statements concerning attitudes, emotional reactions, physical symptoms, psychological symptoms and previous experiences presented in a true/false/cannot say format.

E True

In this test the subject is given a series of standardized sentences to complete.

References/Further Reading

Introduction to Psychology, 8th edn, pp. 404–10.
Revision Notes in Psychiatry, p. 24.

Answers

5.1

The concept of developmental stages in psychology implies that:

- behaviours at a given stage are organized around a dominant theme
- behaviours at one stage are qualitatively different from behaviours that appear at earlier or later stages
- all children go through the same stages in the same order – while environmental factors may alter the speed of development, the order of stages remains the same.

There exist several stage theories focusing variously on, for example:

- cognitive development
- psychosexual development
- moral development
- social development.

A True

Kohlberg's stage theory focuses on moral development.

B False

Charles Spearman (1863–1945) was a British psychologist who developed important advances in statistical science, such as his rank correlation coefficient which could be applied more widely than the Pearson correlation coefficient. Also, using factor analysis, Spearman identified a general factor, g, and a specific factor, s, of intelligence; it was proposed that the level of g was associated with how intelligent the individual was.

C True

Piaget's model focuses on cognitive development.

D True

Sigmund Freud's theory focuses on psychosexual development.

E True

Erikson's model focuses on psychosocial development.

References/Further Reading

Introduction to Psychology, 8th edn, pp. 64–5.
Revision Notes in Psychiatry, pp. 25 and 338.

5.2

A True

Using cuddly and wire artificial surrogate mothers and infant rhesus monkeys, Harlow found that attachment is a function of the requirement to be in contact with a soft object (contact comfort) that provides security.

B True

Lorenz considered attachment to result from imprinting whereby, for example, geese, during a critical period soon after hatching, persistently follow the first nearby moving object encountered.

C False

Tanner described a standardized system for recording breast, pubic hair and genital maturation.

D False

The concept of a transitional object, i.e. an object that is neither oneself nor another person (including mother) and that is selected by an infant between 4 and 18 months of age for self-soothing and anxiety reduction, is associated with Winnicott. Such an object helps during the process of separation–individuation.

E True

Attachment theory comes from the work of Bowlby.

References/Further Reading

Revision Notes in Psychiatry, pp. 25, 26, 36 and 102.

5.3

Attachment refers to the tendency of infants to remain close to certain people (attachment figures) with whom they share strong positive emotional ties and in whose presence they feel more secure. In non-human species, attachment to the mother may manifest in various ways:

• infant monkeys cling to the mother's chest as she moves about
• puppies climb over each other attempting to reach the mother's warm belly
• ducklings and baby chicks follow their mother, making sounds to which she responds and going to her when frightened.

A False

Attachment usually takes place from infant to mother. In contrast, neonatal–maternal bonding takes place in the opposite direction. Both processes can start immediately after birth.

B False

Monotropic attachment refers to the situation in which the attachment is to one individual, usually the mother. Polytropic attachment (i.e. attachment to more than one individual) is less common.

C True

Some behaviourists consider attachment to result from the mother acting as a conditioned reinforcer. However, this theory was challenged by Harlow who, using cuddly and wire artificial surrogate mothers and infant rhesus monkeys, found that attachment is a function of the requirement to be in contact with a soft object (contact comfort), which provides security. Other studies have found that warm or rocking artificial surrogate mothers are preferred to colder or still surrogates respectively.

D False

The attachment process takes an average of 6 months to become fully established.

E True

The mother's attachment behaviour is reinforced by the following behaviours of the infant:

• smiling
• movement
• crying.

References/Further Reading

Introduction to Psychology, 8th edn, pp. 74–80.
Revision Notes in Psychiatry, pp. 25–6.

5.4

After starting to form attachments, around 6 months to 2 years of age, separation from mother leads to the following acute separation reactions:

- first, protest
- second, despair
- finally, detachment.

A True

This manifests in the infant as apathy and misery with an apparent belief that mother may not return.

B False

This refers to those psychological and emotional processes, expressed both internally and externally, that accompany bereavement.

C False

This is one of the stages of bereavement described by Parkes.

D True

The infant is emotionally distant from and indifferent to his or her mother.

E True

The manifestation of protest in the infant includes crying and searching behaviour.

References/Further Reading

Revision Notes in Psychiatry, pp. 26–7, 42.

5.5

Following a failure to form adequate attachments, for example because of prolonged maternal separation or rejecting parents, the effects of maternal deprivation may include:

- developmental language delay
- indiscriminate affection-seeking
- shallow relationships
- enuresis
- aggression
- lack of empathy
- social disinhibition
- attention-seeking and overactivity in school
- poor growth.

A True

This is sometimes referred to as deprivation dwarfism.

B False

C True

D False

A lack of empathy is a recognized feature of maternal deprivation.

E True

References/Further Reading

Revision Notes in Psychiatry, p. 27.

5.6

Dysfunctional families may manifest:

- discord
- overprotection – of the child(ren) by the parents
- rejection – of the child(ren)
- enmeshment
- disengagement
- triangulation
- communication difficulties, e.g. ambiguous or incongruous communications
- myths.

A False

This is a source of error in psychological assessment by interview in which the subject makes a choice of responses that they believe the interviewer desires.

B True

Exclusive alliances are formed within the dysfunctional family, for example between the father and a daughter (although this may, for example, be helpful in preventing the father from leaving home).

C True

The parents may be overinvolved in their children's feelings and lives.

D True

The parents may be underinvolved in their children's feelings and lives.

E True

Myths may be created within dysfunctional families.

References/Further Reading

Revision Notes in Psychiatry, pp. 22 and 28.

5.7

Recognized sequelae of child sexual abuse include:

* anxiety states and anxiety-related symptoms (e.g. sleep disturbance, nightmares, psychosomatic complaints and hypervigilance), re-enactments of the victimization and post-traumatic stress disorder
* depression
* dissociation
* paranoid reactions and mistrust
* excessive reliance on primitive defence mechanisms (e.g. denial, projection, dissociation and splitting)
* borderline personality disorder (especially in women)
* inability to control sexual impulses
* weakened gender identity
* increased incidence of homosexuality
* increased incidence of molesting children (the cycle of abuse may continue – there is a high incidence of sexual abuse in the backgrounds of male and female child molesters)
* drug and alcohol abuse
* eating disorders.

A False

A recognized sequela is an inability to control sexual impulses that may manifest as precocious sexual play with high sexual arousal.

B False

A recognized sequela is weakened gender identity with a tendency for the individual to reject their maleness or femaleness.

C True

D True

E False

A recognized sequela is an increased incidence of homosexuality.

References/Further Reading

Revision Notes in Psychiatry, p. 29.

5.8

Recognized sequelae of physical abuse (which overlap with those of sexual abuse) include:

- anxiety states and anxiety-related symptoms (e.g. sleep disturbance, nightmares, psychosomatic complaints, and hypervigilance), re-enactments of the victimization and post-traumatic stress disorder
- depression
- dissociation
- paranoid reactions and mistrust
- excessive reliance on primitive defence mechanisms (e.g. denial, projection, dissociation and splitting)
- borderline personality disorder (especially in women)
- aggressive and destructive behaviour at home and school
- cognitive and developmental impairment
- delayed language development
- neurological impairment
- abusive behaviour with their own children (the cycle of abuse may continue).

A True

B False

C True

Borderline personality disorder, especially in women, is a recognized sequela.

D True

E True

References/Further Reading

Revision Notes in Psychiatry, pp. 29–30.

5.9

The sensorimotor stage is the first stage of Piaget's model of cognitive development and occurs from birth to 2 years of age.

A True

Circular reactions are repeated voluntary motor activities, for example shaking a toy, occurring from around 2 months. They may be primary, secondary or tertiary:

- primary circular reactions – from 2 to 5 months (approximately), when they have no apparent purpose
- secondary circular reactions – from 5 to 9 months (approximately), when experimentation and purposeful behaviour is gradually manifested
- tertiary circular reactions – from 1 year to 18 months (approximately), include the creation of original behaviour patterns and the purposeful quest for novel experiences.

B False

This is a feature of the concrete operational stage of cognitive development.

C True

Thought processes exhibit egocentrism, in which the infant believes that everything happens in relation to him or her.

D False

In Piaget's model an understanding of the law of conservation of number is said to be normally achieved during the concrete operational stage of cognitive development.

E True

Until around 6 months the infant believes that an object hidden from view no longer exists. Object permanence is fully developed after around the age of 18 months (still in the sensorimotor stage of cognitive development).

References/Further Reading

Revision Notes in Psychiatry, p. 32.

5.10

During the preoperational stage the child learns to use the symbols of language. Thought processes exhibited during this stage include:

* animism
* artificialism
* authoritarian morality
* creationism
* egocentrism
* finalism
* precausal reasoning
* syncretism.

A False

The preoperational stage occurs from age 2 to 7 years.

B True

It is believed by the child during this stage of cognitive development that wrongdoing, including breaking the rules of a game, should be punished according to the degree of the damage caused, whether accidental or not, rather than according to motive; negative events are perceived as punishments.

C False

The preoperational stage is the second stage of Piaget's model of cognitive development.

D True

A teleological approach is taken by the child during this stage of cognitive development in which, for example, stars and the moon exist in order to provide light at night.

E False

The ability systematically to test hypotheses is a feature of the formal operational stage in Piaget's model of cognitive development.

References/Further Reading

Revision Notes in Psychiatry, pp. 32 and 33.

5.11

A False

Language development in normal children up to the age of 3 years is typically as follows:

- in the first hours postnatally, the baby learns to distinguish his or her mother's voice
- by 3–4 months babbling occurs
- by 8 months repetitive babbling occurs
- by 1 year the baby has usually acquired the equivalent designations 'Mama', 'Dada', (no matter what language the parent speaks) and one additional word
- by 18 months a 20- to 50-word vocabulary is expressed in a single word
- by 2 years, two- or three-word utterances can be strung together with some understanding of grammar; these are telegraphic utterances omitting grammatical morphemes (small units of meaning signifying the plural, for example)
- at an average age of 3 years, the child can usually understand a request containing three parts.

B False

Circular reactions are repeated voluntary motor activities, for example shaking a toy, occurring during the sensorimotor stage of cognitive development from around 2 months of age. The age ranges of occurrence of primary, secondary and tertiary circular reactions are approximately as follows:

- primary circular reactions – from 2 to 5 months (approximately)
- secondary circular reactions – from 5 to 9 months (approximately)
- tertiary circular reactions – from 1 year to 18 months (approximately).

C False

This is the fourth of Kohlberg's six developmental stages of moral judgement. Laws and social rules are upheld in order to avoid the censure of authorities and because of guilt about not doing one's duty. Authority orientation is part of level II, i.e. conventional morality, which is the level at which most moral judgements of children lie by the age of 13 years.

D True

A fear of heights typically begins between the ages of 6 to 8 months, and becomes worse when walking starts.

E False

The anal phase of psychosexual development occurs from around 15–18 months to 30–36 months of age. Sigmund Freud believed that during this phase erotogenic pleasure is derived from stimulation of the anal mucosa, initially through faecal excretion, and later also through faecal retention.

References/Further Reading

Revision Notes in Psychiatry, pp. 32–5, 99.

5.12

A False

Early language development in girls is slightly greater than in boys.

B True

Being a twin is associated with slower speech development.

C True

Prolonged second-stage labour is associated with slower language development.

D True

Larger family size is associated with slower speech development.

E False

A bilingual home is not a disadvantage unless there is another cause of slowed language development.

References/Further Reading

Revision Notes in Psychiatry, p. 33.

5.13

Kohlberg presented a set of stories, each containing a moral dilemma, to various individuals of various ages and backgrounds. Questions were posed concerning the moral dilemmas. On the basis of the reasons given for the answers Kohlberg formulated a theory of moral development consisting of six developmental stages of moral judgement categorized into three levels (I–III).

A False

The three levels are:

- preconventional morality (level I)
- conventional morality (level II)
- post-conventional morality (level III).

B False

Reward orientation, in which rules are conformed to in order to be rewarded, is stage 2 and is in level I (preconventional morality).

C True

This is stage 3 and is part of level II. Rules are conformed to in order to avoid the disapproval of others.

D False

Each level has two stages, as follows:

Level I
- Stage 1 – punishment orientation
- Stage 2 – reward orientation.

Level II
- Stage 3 – good-boy/good-girl orientation
- Stage 4 – authority orientation.

Level III
- Stage 5 – social contract orientation
- Stage 6 – ethical principle orientation.

E False

The age ranges during which each level typically occurs are as follows:

- Level I – this is the level at which the moral judgements of children up to the age of 7 years mainly lie
- Level II – this is the level at which most moral judgements of children lie by the age of 13 years
- Level III – this level, which may never be reached even in adulthood, requires individuals to have achieved the later stages of Piaget's formal operational stage.

References/Further Reading

Introduction to Psychology, 8th edn, pp. 81–3.
Revision Notes in Psychiatry, pp. 33–4.

5.14

The types of fear that develop in childhood and adolescence differ with age as follows:

- 6 months – fear of novel stimuli begins (such as fear of strangers), reaching a peak at 18 months to 2 years
- 6–8 months – fear of heights begins, and becomes worse when walking starts
- 3–5 years – common fears are those of animals, the dark and 'monsters'
- 6–11 years – fear of shameful social situations (such as ridicule) begins
- adolescence – fear of death, failure, social gatherings (such as parties) and thermonuclear war may be particularly evident.

A False

B True

C False

D False

E True

References/Further Reading

Revision Notes in Psychiatry, p. 35.

5.15

Sex determination is primarily as a result of the sex chromosomes (XX female and XY male). Gonad formation is first indicated in the embryo by the appearance of an area of thickened epithelium on the medial aspect of the mesonephric ridge during week 5. Factors affecting subsequent differentiation of the genital organs into male ones (epididymis, ductus (vas) deferens, ejaculatory ducts, penis and scrotum) or female ones (fallopian tubes, uterus, clitoris and vagina) during ontogeny include:

- the Y chromosome
- the degree of ripeness of the ovum at fertilization
- endocrine actions.

A True

In mammals, testis determination is under the control of the testis-determining factor borne by the Y chromosome. SRY, a gene cloned from the sex-determining region of the human Y chromosome, has been equated with the testis-determining factor in humans.

B True

Over-ripeness of the ovum at fertilization is associated with a reduced number of primordial germ cells. This in turn leads to a masculinizing effect on genetic women.

C True

21-Hydroxylase deficiency is the commonest subtype of congenital adrenal hyperplasia and is caused by an abnormality near the HLA-B and HLA-D loci on 6p21.3 that causes a cytochrome P450 enzyme abnormality. 21-Hydroxylase deficiency can lead to a masculinizing effect on a genetically female fetus, which may be born with either ambiguous or male genitalia.

D False

A genetically male fetus with testes may develop female genitalia in the absence of fetal androgen.

E True

See **B** above.

References/Further Reading

Revision Notes in Psychiatry, pp. 35–7.

5.16

Puberty consists of a series of physical and physiological changes that convert a child into an adult who is capable of sexual reproduction. The physical changes include:

- growth spurt
- change in body proportion
- development of sexual organs
- development of secondary sexual characteristics.

A True

A raising of the threshold for gonadohypothalamic negative feedback precedes the onset of puberty. An increase in adrenal (suprarenal) androgen release usually begins between the ages of 6 and 8 years in both men and women and continues until 13–15 years. This phenomenon is known as adrenarche and is characterized by an increase in dehydroepiandosterone, dehydroepiandosterone sulphate and androstenedione. The only clear somatic function of these adrenal androgens appears to be the promotion of pubic and axillary hair growth. The adolescent growth spurt does not depend on them.

B False

In 95% of girls the onset of puberty occurs between 9 and 13 years. The first sign is:

- breast formation – in 80%
- pubic hair growth – in 20%.

In Western countries, menarche occurs at a mean age of 13.5 years.

C False

In 95% of boys the onset of puberty occurs between 9.5 and 13.5 years. The first sign is usually testicular and scrotal enlargement, followed by growth of the penis and pubic hair. On average, the first ejaculation occurs at around 13 years.

D True

Tanner described a standardized system for recording breast, pubic hair and genital maturation.

E False

There is a failure at puberty to develop normal secondary sex characteristics in Turner's syndrome; pubic hair development is scant.

References/Further Reading

Revision Notes in Psychiatry, p. 36.
Essential Reproduction, 4th edn, pp. 111–14.

5.17

A False

Gender identity is an individual's perception and self-awareness with respect to gender. Gender role is the type of behaviour that an individual engages in that identifies him or her as being male or female, for example with respect to the type of clothes worn and the use of cosmetics.

B False

Gender identity is usually established by the age of 3–4 years and usually remains firmly established thereafter.

C True

See **B** above.

D True

Gender typing or sex typing is the process by which individuals acquire a sense of gender and gender-related cultural traits appropriate to the society and age into which they are born.

E True

Parents play a major role in sex typing. They serve as the child's first models of male and female behaviour. Their attitudes towards their own sex roles and the way they interact with each other influence the child's views. Further, parents shape sex-typed behaviour directly in many other ways, such as:

- the toys provided
- the activities encouraged
- their responses to behaviours considered appropriate or inappropriate to the child's gender
- how the child is dressed.

References/Further Reading

Introduction to Psychology, 8th edn, pp. 87–92.
Revision Notes in Psychiatry, p. 36.

5.18

Offer and Offer (1975) showed that, in general, adolescence is a time of less turmoil and upheaval than previously thought. They studied a cohort of American men who had been aged 14 years in 1962. Sixty-one of these adolescents were studied intensively and followed-up into adulthood.

A False

There were no serious drug problems among the adolescents.

B False

The adolescents showed no significant difference in basic values from those of their parents.

C True

The adolescents came mainly from intact families.

D False

There was no major delinquent activity among the adolescents.

E True

Seventy-four per cent of the adolescents went to college during the first year after high school graduation.

References/Further Reading

Offer, B. and Offer, J.B. (1975) *From Teenage to Young Manhood: A Psychological Study.* New York: Basic Books.
Revision Notes in Psychiatry, p. 40.

5.19

Offer and Offer (1975) identified the following three adolescent developmental routes (the percentages given are those of the sample of adolescents they studied; the remaining 21% could not be classified easily, but were closer to the first two categories than to the third one):

- continuous growth (23%)
- surgent growth (35%)
- tumultuous growth (21%).

A False

B True

Eriksonian intimacy was achieved and shame and guilt could be displayed. Major separation, death and severe illness were less frequent. Their parents encouraged independence.

C False

A group of ego-resilient adolescents was identified by Block and Haan (1971) using factor analysis in a cohort of 84 male adolescents studied longitudinally to adulthood. Other groups isolated in this cohort of male adolescents included:

- belated adjustors – similar to the surgent group of Offer and Offer
- vulnerable overcontrollers
- anomic extroverts – less inner life and relatively uncertain values
- unsettled undercontrollers – given to impulsivity.

D True

The adolescents in this group were 'late-bloomers'. They were more likely than the first group to have frequent depressive and anxious moments. Although often successful, they were less introspective and not as action-oriented as the first group. There were more areas of disagreement with their parents.

E True

Recurrent self-doubt and conflict with their families occurred in this group. Their backgrounds were less stable than in the first two groups. The arts, humanities and social sciences were preferred to professional and business careers.

References/Further Reading

Block, J. and Haan, N. (1971) *Lives Through Time*. Berkeley, CA: Bancroft Books.
Offer, B. and Offer, J.B. (1975) *From Teenage to Young Manhood: A Psychological Study*. New York: Basic Books.
Revision Notes in Psychiatry, p. 40.

5.20

Using factor analysis in a cohort of 86 female adolescents studied longitudinally to adulthood, Block and Haan (1971) identified the following groups:

- female prototype
- cognitive type
- hyperfeminine repressors
- dominating narcissists
- vulnerable undercontrollers
- lonely independents.

A True

Individuals in this group tended to be intellectualized in the way that problems were negotiated.

B False

A group of belated adjustors was identified by Block and Haan (1971) among adolescent men. They were similar to the surgent group of Offer and Offer (1975).

C True

This group was similar to hysterical personality disorder.

D True

E True

References/Further Reading

Block, J. and Haan, N. (1971) *Lives Through Time*. Berkeley, CA: Bancroft Books.
Offer, B. and Offer, J.B. (1975) *From Teenage to Young Manhood: A Psychological Study*. New York: Basic Books.
Revision Notes in Psychiatry, pp. 40–1.

5.21

Grief refers to those psychological and emotional processes, expressed both internally and externally, that accompany bereavement. The symptomatology of normal grief may include:

- initial shock and disbelief – 'a feeling of numbness'
- increasing awareness of the loss is associated with painful emotions of sadness and anger
- anger may be denied
- irritability
- somatic distress
- identification phenomena.

The diagnosis of Major Depressive Disorder in DSM-IV is generally not given unless the symptoms are still present two months after the loss. However, the presence of certain symptoms that are not characteristic of a normal grief reaction may be helpful in differentiating bereavement from a Major Depressive Episode:

- guilt about things other than actions taken or not taken by the survivor at the time of the death
- thoughts of death other than the survivor feeling that he or she would be better off dead or should have died with the deceased person
- morbid preoccupation with worthlessness
- marked psychomotor retardation
- prolonged and marked functional impairment
- hallucinatory experiences other than thinking that he or she hears the voice of, or transiently sees the image of, the deceased person.

A True

B False

C True

D True

E False

References/Further Reading

Revision Notes in Psychiatry, pp. 42–3.

5.22

The symptomatology of normal grief is given in the answer to the previous question. In 1944 Lindemann read to the centenary meeting of the American Psychiatric Association the results of his study of 101 bereaved individuals, many of whom had lost loved ones in the tragic Cocoanut Grove nightclub fire in Boston, MA, USA. He identified the following five points as being pathognomonic of acute grief:

- somatic distress
- preoccupation with the image of the deceased
- guilt
- hostile reactions
- loss of patterns of conduct.

Lindemann described the following morbid grief reactions:

- delay of reaction
- distorted reactions, which are subclassified into
  - overactivity without a sense of loss
  - the acquisition of symptoms belonging to the last illness of the deceased
  - a recognized medical disease
  - alteration in relationship to friends and relatives
  - furious hostility against specific persons
  - loss of affectivity
  - a lasting loss of patterns of social interaction
  - activities attain a colouring detrimental to social and economic existence
  - agitated depression.

A False

This is a feature of normal grief.

B False

This is a feature of normal grief as are other manifestations of somatic distress such as:

- sleep disturbance
- tearfulness
- loss of appetite
- weight loss
- loss of libido
- anhedonia.

C False

Identification phenomena, in which the mannerisms and characteristics of the deceased may be taken on, may be a feature of normal grief.

D True

E False

In a morbid grief reaction, a furious hostility against specific persons may occur, whereas in normal grief anger may be denied.

References/Further Reading

Revision Notes in Psychiatry, pp. 42–3.

6 PRINCIPLES OF EVALUATION AND PSYCHOMETRICS

Answers

6.1

As these are working adults, the social classes included in this variable are from I to V Inclusive; 0 is not included.

A False

Qualitative variables refer to attributes that can be categorized such that the categories do not have a numerical relationship with each other. Examples include eye colour, hair colour and religious affiliation. Quantitative variables, on the other hand, refer to numerically represented data. In this case, social class is categorized such that the categories (1–5) have a numerical relationship with each other, and therefore the variable is quantitative. The variable takes values from 1 to 5.

B False

Characteristic properties of interval measurement scales are:

- Categories are mutually exclusive.
- Categories are logically ordered.
- There is an equal distance between adjacent categories.

While the first two of these properties clearly apply to the variable in this question, the third property does not. It is not the case that, for instance, the 'difference' (whatever that might mean) between social classes 1 and 2 is the same as the 'difference' between social classes 2 and 3. Note that the second property does apply as it is the case that:

social class 1 > social class 2 > social class 3 > social class 4 > social class 5

Hence this variable is ordinal.

C True

Discrete quantitative variables can only take on known fixed values. In this case the variable concerned can only theoretically take on the values 1, 2, 3, 4 or 5. (In practice there may be an additional value for 'other' or 'missing'.) In contrast, a continuous quantitative variable can take on any value in a defined range; however, if we define the range of values that the variable in this question can take as being from 1 to 5, then clearly a non-integer value of the social class for an individual, such as 1.3 say, is meaningless.

D True

The values are: 1, 2, 3, 4, 5 ± other/missing.

E False

References/Further Reading

Revision Notes in Psychiatry, pp. 48–9.

6.2

Characteristic properties of ratio measurement scales are

- Categories are mutually exclusive.
- Categories are logically ordered.
- There is an equal distance between adjacent categories.
- There is a true zero point.

A False

B False

The Centigrade temperature scale does not have a true zero point. 0 °C is, so far as absolute temperature is concerned, an arbitrary point. Thus 40 °C, for example, does not represent a temperature that is twice as hot as 20 °C. The Kelvin temperature scale, on the other hand, does have a true zero point and therefore temperatures expressed in Kelvin are measured on a ratio scale.

C True

D True

E False

This is a nominal variable for which only the first of the above characteristic properties applies.

References/Further Reading

Revision Notes in Psychiatry, p. 49.

6.3

A False

B True

Periodic sampling is a type of systematic sampling in which every nth member of the population is chosen. This may not always lead to a random choice because of an unforeseen underlying pattern.

C True

Stratified sampling is a type of systematic sampling in which a given population is stratified before samples are chosen from each stratum. This can be useful when studying a disease that varies with respect to sex and age, for example.

D True

Compared with simple random sampling, systematic sampling saves time and effort.

E True

A simple random sample is one chosen from a given population such that every possible sample of the same size has the same probability of being chosen.

References/Further Reading

Revision Notes in Psychiatry, p. 48.

6.4

A True

The chi-squared distribution is a continuous asymmetrical probability distribution. The chi-squared distribution with v degrees of freedom, $\chi^2(v)$, is obtained from the sum of the squares of v independent variables, Z_1 to Z_v, where each $Z \sim N(0, 1)$:

If $W = \sum Z_i^2$, where $i = 1$ to v, and $Z_i \sim N(0, 1)$

Then $W \sim \chi^2(v)$

B False

The Bernoulli distribution is the probability distribution for a discrete binary variable (range = 0, 1), which is a special case of the binomial distribution, $B(1, p)$, where p is the probability of 'success':

mean = p

variance = $p(1 - p)$

It is named after James Bernoulli, who lived from 1654 to 1705.

C False

The binomial distribution, $B(n, p)$, is the probability distribution for a discrete finite variable (range = 0, 1, 2,..., n):

mean = np

variance = $np(1 - p)$

D True

The normal distribution, $N(\mu, \sigma^2)$, is the probability distribution for a continuous variable (range = $\Re$):

mean = μ

variance = σ^2

E True

The F distribution is related to the χ^2 distribution and is an asymmetrical continuous probability distribution. A given F distribution is described in terms of v_1 and v_2, each of which gives a number of degrees of freedom. This is usually abbreviated to $F(v_1, v_2)$.

References/Further Reading

Revision Notes in Psychiatry, pp. 49–51.

6.5

A True

The median is equal to the mean in a normal distribution, which is given as 100 in this case.

B False

The variance is the square of the standard deviation. As the standard deviation is given as 15, the variance cannot equal 15.

C False

The total area under the probability density function curve is 1.

D False

The mode is equal to the mean in a normal distribution, which is given as 100 in this case.

E True

The interval from 85 to 115 (inclusive) represents:

$$(100 - 15) \text{ to } (100 + 15)$$

i.e. (mean – standard deviation) to (mean + standard deviation)

The interval 1 standard deviation either side of the mean of the probability density function of a normal distribution encloses 68.27% of the total area under the curve.

References/Further Reading

Revision Notes in Psychiatry, pp. 50 and 52.

6.6

Properties of the normal distribution probability density function curve include:

- It is unimodal.
- It is continuous.
- It is symmetrical about its mean.
- Its mean, median and mode are all equal.
- The area under the curve is 1.
- The curve tends to zero as the variable moves in either direction from the mean.

The interval 1 standard deviation either side of the mean of the probability density function of a normal distribution encloses 68.27% of the total area under the curve.

The interval 2 standard deviations either side of the mean of the probability density function of a normal distribution encloses 95.45% of the total area under the curve.

The interval 3 standard deviations either side of the mean of the probability density function of a normal distribution encloses 99.73% of the total area under the curve.

A False

B True

C False

The interval (mean – 2 standard deviations) to (mean + 2 standard deviations) encloses 95.45% of the total area under the curve (see above). Hence, as the normal distribution probability density function curve is symmetrical about its mean, it follows that the interval mean to (mean + 2 standard deviations) encloses (95.45/2)% of the total area under the curve.

D True

For $N(\mu, \sigma^2)$ the two-tailed 5% points are given by:

$$\mu - 1.96\sigma$$

$$\mu + 1.96\sigma$$

E True

When $n < 30$, the t distribution, $t(v)$ or t_v, is used in making inferences about the mean of a normal population when its variance is unknown. The t distribution is symmetrical about the mean but has longer tails than the standard normal distribution.

v is the number of degrees of freedom, and is given by:

$$v = n - 1$$

The standard normal distribution is the normal distribution with mean = 0 and variance = 1, i.e. $N(0,1)$.

For $n \geq 30$, $t(v) \approx N(0, 1)$.

References/Further Reading

Revision Notes in Psychiatry, pp. 50–1.

6.7

A True

The (arithmetic) mean (or average) of a sample with n items $(x_1, x_2, x_3, \ldots, x_n)$, $\bar{x}$, is given by:

$\bar{x} = (\Sigma x)/n$

In this case

$\Sigma x = 4 + 8 + 8 + 10 = 30$

$n = 4$ (because there are four items)

Therefore, omitting units, the mean is given by

$(\Sigma x)/n = 30/4 = 7.5$

The correct units are those of x, i.e. years, and so the mean is 7.5 years.

B False

The median is the middle value of a set of observations ranked in order. If the number of observations is odd:

median = middle value

If the number of observations is even:

median = arithmetic mean of the two middle values

In this case the number of observations is four, which is even. The two middle values, when the observations are ranked in order, are 8 and 8. Hence, omitting units, the median is given by:

median = arithmetic mean of 8 and 8 = 8

The correct units are those of the observations, i.e. years, and so the median is 8 years.

C True

The mode of a distribution is the value of the observation occurring most frequently. In this case the mode is 8 years.

D False

No calculations are required to answer this. Note instead that whereas the standard deviation of a distribution is based on deviations from the mean and has the same units as the original observations, the variance is the square of the standard deviation and has units that are the square of those of the observations. Therefore the units of the variance in this case should be y^2, year^2 or squared years. As the units given (years) are incorrect, the answer must be false.

E True

The range is the difference between the smallest and largest values in a distribution:

range = largest value – smallest value

Therefore, omitting units, the range is given by

largest value – smallest value

$= 10 - 4 = 6$

The correct units are those of the observations, i.e. years, and so the range is 6 years.

References/Further Reading

Revision Notes in Psychiatry, pp. 51–2.

6.8

Outliers are extreme values.

A True

Graphical methods such as scatterplots and boxplots may allow visual identification of possible outliers.

B False

Outliers can exert an extreme effect on the arithmetic mean, particularly when the total number of values is small. The median is less affected in such a case and may therefore be preferred as a measure of central tendency.

C False

As the range is the difference between the largest and smallest values in a distribution, it follows that the range is always affected by the presence of outliers. Hence outliers are said to exert an extreme effect on the range. Measures of dispersion relating to quantiles are less affected in such a case and may therefore be preferred. Because it takes into account all the values in a distribution, the standard deviation (or variance) may be affected by outliers, although less so than the range.

D True

Outliers may exert an extreme effect on the results of correlation and linear regression. In such cases it may be necessary to consider excluding outliers from the calculations.

E True

See **D** above.

References/Further Reading

Revision Notes in Psychiatry, p. 54.

6.9

Boxplots can be used to represent a continuous variable. A boxplot consists of a box whose longer sides are usually placed vertically, with vertical lines (whiskers) extending vertically. However, this arrangement is sometimes represented horizontally (the whole plot being rotated clockwise through an angle of 90°) if more convenient.

A True

Boxplots can be useful for comparing two or more sets of observations diagrammatically, before or in addition to more formal statistical analyses.

B False

The length of the box is the interquartile range.

C False

The upper boundary of the box is the upper (third) quartile.

D False

The horizontal line inside the box is the median (second quartile). This is often, though not necessarily, a thick line.

E False

They are also known as box-and-whisker plots. Stem-and-leaf plots can also be used to represent a continuous variable. The stems in such plots consist of a vertical column of numbers on the left-hand side of the plot. The leaves are numbers to the right of the stems, which may, for example, represent tenths. All the individual data can then be derived by combining the individual leaves with their corresponding stems, while the shape of the overall plot indicates the shape of the distribution. Stem-and-leaf plots are particularly easy to represent in computer printouts. For instance, the distribution 13.5, 13.7, 14.5, 14.6, 14.6, 14.7, 15.2, 15.9 and 16.4 (arbitrary units) may be represented as the following stem-and-leaf plot:

13	5 7
14	5 6 6 7
15	2 9
16	4

References/Further Reading

Revision Notes in Psychiatry, pp. 54–5.

6.10

Descriptive statistics are ways of organizing and describing data. Examples include:

- diagrams
- graphical representations
- numerical representations
- tables.

A True

B True

C False

Inferential statistics allow conclusions to be inferred from data. A *P*-value is an inferential statistic.

D False

A confidence interval is an inferential statistic.

E True

References/Further Reading

Revision Notes in Psychiatry, pp. 55–6.

6.11

The initial hypothesis is the null hypothesis, H_0, usually representing no change:

$$H_0: \theta = \theta_0$$

where θ is the unknown parameter and θ_0 is its hypothesized value. A composite hypothesis is one involving more than one value for the population parameter.

A False

B False

C True

A two-sided significance test is a hypothesis test involving a composite alternative hypothesis of the following type

$$H_1: \theta \neq \theta_0$$

D True

A one-sided significance test is a hypothesis test involving a composite alternative hypothesis of the following types

$$H_1: \theta > \theta_0$$

$$H_1: \theta < \theta_0$$

E True
See **D** above.

References/Further Reading

Revision Notes in Psychiatry, pp. 55–6.

6.12

A False

The 95% confidence interval for the difference includes zero.

B True

As this is a 95% confidence interval, the value of α, the significance level, is 5% or 0.05. The significance level, α, is the size of the critical region and represents the following probability:

$$\alpha = P(\text{type I error})$$

where a type I error is the error of wrongly rejecting the null hypothesis (H_0) when it is true.

C False

This statement is incorrect. The correct meaning of a 95% confidence interval is as follows. If a 95% confidence interval from a statistic (or statistics) is calculated, this implies that, if the study were repeated with other random samples taken from the same parent population(s) and further 95% confidence intervals similarly individually calculated, then the overall proportion of these confidence intervals that included the corresponding population parameter(s) would tend to 95%.

D True

This is true at the 5% level of significance, because the 95% confidence interval for the difference includes zero.

E False

A one-sided confidence interval is not the same as half a two-sided confidence interval starting (or ending) at zero.

References/Further Reading

Revision Notes in Psychiatry, pp. 56–7.

6.13

A False

The data are not paired but, rather, consist of two independent samples. However, an independent samples t-test could be used here. This procedure tests the null hypothesis that the data are a sample from a population in which the mean of a test variable is equal in two independent (unrelated) groups of cases. Assuming equal population variances (which can be checked using Levene's test), the standard error of the difference between two means, $\bar{x}_1$ and $\bar{x}_2$, of two independent samples (taken from the same parent population) of respective sizes n_1 and n_2, and respective standard deviations s_1 and s_2, $(s_1 \approx s_2)$ is given by:

$$\text{standard error of difference} = s\sqrt{[1/n_1 + 1/n_2]}$$

where the pooled standard deviation s is given by:

$$s = \sqrt{\{[(n_1 - 1)s_1^2 + (n_2 - 1)s_2^2]/(n_1 + n_2 - 2)\}}$$

If the population variances cannot be assumed to be equal, then the standard error is given by

$$\text{standard error of difference} = \sqrt{[s_1^2/n_1 + s_2^2/n_2]}$$

B False

The chi-squared (χ^2) test can be used to compare independent qualitative and discrete quantitative variables presented in the form of contingency tables containing the data frequencies.

C True

The two-sample t-test is simply a special case of the one-way analysis of variance (ANOVA) model. The one-way ANOVA model applies to a single categorical explanatory variable (in this case the grouping of the subjects – schizophrenic or normal control) and a continuous response variable (in this case the haemoglobin level), and postulates that the response (haemoglobin level) of the ith experimental unit for the jth value of the categorical explanatory variable is given by:

$$Y_{ij} = \mu_j + \varepsilon_{ij}$$

where each $\varepsilon_{ij} \sim N(0, \sigma^2)$ and all the ε_{ij} values are independent of one another. The overall result of applying a one-way ANOVA test in this case would be exactly the same as that obtained from the application of the independent sample t-test.

D True

This is a non-parametric alternative to the independent samples t-test. The test statistic, U, is the smaller of U_1 and U_2:

$$U_1 = n_1 n_2 + \tfrac{1}{2} n_1(n_1 + 1) - R_1$$
$$U_2 = n_1 n_2 + \tfrac{1}{2} n_2(n_2 + 1) - R_2$$

where n_1 = number of observations in the first group; n_2 = number of observations in the second group; R_1 = sum of the ranks assigned to the first group; R_2 = sum of the ranks assigned to the second group.

For $n_1 \geq 8$ and $n_2 \geq 8$, $U \sim N(\mu, \sigma^2)$, where

$$\mu = n_1 n_2/2$$

$$\sigma^2 = n_1 n_2(n_1 + n_2 + 1)/12$$

E False

This is a test of equality of variances and can be used, for example, as part of an independent samples *t*-test (see the answer to A above).

References/Further Reading

Revision Notes in Psychiatry, pp. 57–9.

6.14

The chi-squared (χ^2) test is a test that can be used to compare independent qualitative and discrete variables presented in the form of contingency tables containing the data frequencies.

Null hypothesis
For a given contingency table, under H_0,

   expected value of a cell = row total × column total/sum of cells

Calculation of χ^2
The value of χ^2 for a contingency table is calculated from

   $\chi^2 \Sigma[(O - E)^2/E]$

where O = observed value, E = expected value.

A False

It is a non-parametric test.

B True

If the overall total in the contingency table is between 20 and 100, then a better fit with the continuous χ^2 distribution is provided by using Yates' continuity correction.

C False

Fisher's exact probability test allows the calculation of exact prababilities only for 2 × 2 contingency tables.

D False

In order to use the χ^2 distribution, the number of degress of freedom of a contingency table, v, is given by

   $v = (r - 1)(k - 1)$

where r = number of rows, k = number of columns.

   In this case, $r = 3$ and $k = 3$. Therefore, the number of degrees of freedom is given by

   $(r - 1)(k - 1)$
   $= (3 - 1)(3 - 1)$
   $= 2 \times 2$
   $= 4$

E False

For a contingency table with more than 1 degree of freedom, the following criteria should be fulfilled for the test to be valid:

- each expected value ≥ 1
- in at least 80% of cases, expected value > 5

References/Further Reading

Revision Notes in Psychiatry, pp. 58–9.

6.15

Clinical trials are planned experiments carried out on humans to assess the effectiveness of different forms of treatment. The following classification of clinical trials is used by the pharmaceutical industry:

- phase I trial – clinical pharmacology and toxicity
- phase II trial – initial clinical investigation
- phase III trial – full-scale treatment evaluation
- phase IV trial – post-marketing surveillance.

A True

The gold standard of clinical trials is the randomized double-blind controlled trial in which:

- Allocation of treatments to subjects is randomized.
- Each subject does not know which treatment has been received by him/her.
- The investigator(s) do not know the treatment allocation before the end of the trial.

B True

C False

They are carried out in phase I trials.

D False

E True

References/Further Reading

Revision Notes in Psychiatry, p. 61.

6.16

Psychological concepts such as attitude and intelligence are considered to be latent traits or hypothetical constructs that are believed to exist. Although not directly observable, constructs can be used to explain phenomena that can be observed and to make predictions. In the development and use of psychometric tests, in particular, factor analysis may be used to identify factors, corresponding to latent traits or hypothetical constructs, that may account for correlations observed between the scores on tests or subtests for a large sample of subjects.

A False

B True

C True

D True

E True

References/Further Reading

Revision Notes in Psychiatry, p. 63.

6.17

A False

The reliability of a test or measuring instrument describes the level of agreement between repeated measurements. It is the validity of a test or measuring instrument that is the term used to describe whether it measures what it purports to measure.

B True

Reliability can be expressed as the ratio of the variance of the true scores to the variance of the observed scores:

$$\text{reliability} = \sigma_t^2 /(\sigma_t^2 + \sigma_e^2)$$

where

σ_t^2 = true score variance

σ_e^2 = measurement error variance

C False

With the definition given in part B above, the range of values that the reliability can take is given by:

$$0 \leq \text{reliability} \leq 1$$

A low value, close to zero, implies low reliability, while a high value, close to 1, implies high reliability.

D True

Alternative forms reliability describes the level of agreement between assessments of the same material by two supposedly similar forms of the test or measuring instrument made either at the same time or immediately one after the other.

E True

Split-half reliability describes the level of agreement between assessments by two halves of a split test or measuring instrument of the same material made under similar circumstances. As some tests or measuring instruments contain different sections measuring different aspects, in such cases it may be appropriate to create the halves by using alternative questions, thereby maintaining the balance of each half.

References/Further Reading

Revision Notes in Psychiatry, pp. 63–5.

6.18

A True

Measuring the percentage agreement is the simplest but most unsatisfactory method of assessing the reliability, because it does not take into account agreement between observers owing to chance.

B True

The product-moment correlation coefficient, r, may give spuriously high results, particularly if there is chance agreement of many values. It may even give the maximum value of 1 for the agreement between two raters, even if they do not agree at all – if, for example, one of the raters consistently rates scores on the test or measuring instrument at twice the values rated by the other rater.

C True

The kappa statistic, or kappa coefficient, κ, is a measure of agreement in which allowance is made for chance agreement. It is most appropriate when different categories of measurement are being recorded and is calculated from the following formula:

$$\kappa = (P_o - P_c)/(1 - P_c)$$

where

P_c = the chance agreement, P_o = observed proportion of agreement.

The range of values that κ can take is:

$\kappa = 1$ (complete agreement)

$0 < \kappa < 1$ (observed agreement > chance agreement)

$\kappa = 0$ (observed agreement = chance agreement)

$\kappa < 0$ (observed agreement < chance agreement)

The weighted kappa, κ_w, is a version of κ that takes into account differences in the seriousness of disagreements (represented by the weightings).

D True

The intraclass correlation coefficient, r_i, is more appropriate than κ or r if agreement is being measured for several items that can be regarded as part of a continuum or dimension. For two raters, the value of r_i is derived from the corresponding value of r:

$$r_i = \{[\Sigma(s_1^2 + s_2^2) - (s_1 - s_2)^2]r - (\bar{x}_1 - \bar{x}_2)^2/2\}/\{(s_1^2 + s_2^2) + (\bar{x}_1 - \bar{x}_2)^2/2\}$$

where

r = the product-moment correlation coefficient between the scores of the two raters
s_1 = the standard deviation of the scores for the first rater
s_2 = the standard deviation of the scores for the second rater
$\bar{x}_1$ = the mean of the scores for the first rater
$\bar{x}_2$ = the mean of the scores for the second rater

It follows that:

if $\bar{x}_1 = \bar{x}_2$ and $s_1 = s_2$

then $r_i = r$

else $r_i < r$

For more than two raters, the value of r_i is derived from the corresponding two-way ANOVA for (raters × subjects):

$$r_i = n_s(s_{ms} - e_{ms})/\{n_s s_{ms} + n_r\ r_{ms} + (n_s n_r - n_s - n_r)e_{ms}\}$$

where

n_r = number of raters
n_s = number of subjects
e_{ms} = errors mean square
r_{ms} = raters mean square
s_{ms} = subjects mean square

E True

Cronbach's alpha, α, gives a measure of the average correlation between all the items when assessing split-half reliability. It thereby indicates the internal consistency of the test or measuring instrument.

References/Further Reading

Revision Notes in Psychiatry, pp. 64–5.

6.19

The validity of a test or measuring instrument is the term used to describe whether it measures what it purports to measure. Types include:

- content validity
- predictive validity
- concurrent validity
- criterion validity
- incremental validity
- cross-validity
- convergent validity
- divergent validity
- construct validity.

A True

Content validity examines whether the specific measurements aimed for by the test or measuring instrument are assessing the content of the measurement in question.

B True

Predictive validity determines the extent of agreement between a present measurement and one in the future.

C False

Face validity is the subjective judgement as to whether a test or measuring instrument appears on the surface to measure the feature in question. In spite of its name it is not strictly a type of validity and so, strictly speaking, the answer should be False.

D False

E True

Convergent validity is established when measures expected to be correlated, since they measure the same phenomena, are indeed found to be associated, while divergent validity is established when measures discriminate successfully between other measures of unrelated constructs. Construct validity is determined by establishing both convergent and divergent validity, and is closely connected with the theoretical rationale underpinning the test or measuring instrument. It involves showing the power of the hypothetical construct(s) or latent traits both to explain observations and to make predictions.

References/Further Reading

Revision Notes in Psychiatry, pp. 65–6.

6.20

A False

A type II error is the error of wrongly accepting the null hypothesis, H_0, when it is false. The probability of making a type II error is denoted by β

$\beta = P(\text{type II error})$

The description given in the question is that of power. The power of a test is the probability that the null hypothesis, H_0, is rejected when it is indeed false. It is related to β, the probability of making a type II error, in the following way:

power $= 1 - \beta$

B False

A type I error is the error of wrongly rejecting the null hypothesis, H_0, when it is true.

C True

The probability of making a type I error is denoted by α, the significance level:

$\alpha = P(\text{type I error})$

D False

The specificity of a test or measuring instrument is the proportion of negative results/cases correctly identified:

specificity = (true negative)/(true negative + false positive)

This ratio needs to be multiplied by 100 if the sensitivity is to be given as a percentage. In contrast, the sensitivity of a test or measuring instrument is the proportion of positive results/cases correctly identified:

sensitivity = (true positive)/(true positive + false negative)

Again, this ratio needs to be multiplied by 100 if the sensitivity is to be given as a percentage.

E True

The predictive value of a negative result from a research measure is the proportion of the negative results that is true negative:

predictive value of a negative result = (true negative)/(true negative + false negative)

Similarly, the predictive value of a positive result from a research measure is the proportion of the positive results that is true positive:

predictive value of a positive result = (true positive)/(true positive + false positive)

References/Further Reading

Revision Notes in Psychiatry, pp. 66–7.

6.21

Types of bias include:

- selection bias
- observer bias
- recall bias
- information bias
- confounding bias.

A True

In epidemiological studies, recall bias occurs when there is a difference in knowledge between the subjects in the case and in the comparison groups, leading to a biased recall. For example, in case–control studies, the knowledge on the part of subjects (or, in the case of childhood disorders, their parents) as to whether or not they have a given disorder may bias their recall of exposure to putative risk factors.

B False

This is a type of validity. Convergent validity is established when measures expected to be correlated, because they measure the same phenomena, are indeed found to be associated.

C True

Selection bias occurs when a characteristic associated with the variable(s) of interest leads to higher or lower participation in the research study, such as an epidemiological cross-sectional survey.

D False

This is a type of validity. Concurrent validity compares the measure being assessed with an external valid yardstick at the same time.

E True

Information bias includes both observer bias and recall bias.

References/Further Reading

Revision Notes in Psychiatry, pp. 65–7.

6.22

A False

The term meta-analysis is used to describe the process of evaluating and statistically combining results from two or more existing independent randomized clinical trials addressing similar questions in order to give an overall assessment. It is factor analysis that is an attempt to express a set of multivariate data as a linear function of unobserved, underlying dimensions, or (common) factors together with error terms (specific factors); the common factors associated with each observed variable have individual loadings.

B True

Trials showing a statistically significant difference are more likely to be published than those not finding a statistically significant result. Other difficulties associated with meta-analysis include:

- Researchers finding 'non-significant' results may be less likely to write up their results formally for publication.
- Arriving at selection criteria to determine which studies to include and which not to include in the meta-analysis.
- The different centres in which the different clinical trials have taken place may differ with respect to important variables in such a way as seriously to question the validity of combining their data.
- If the meta-analysis is of clinical trials carried out on widely differing population groups, to whom can the results of the meta-analysis be properly applied?

C True

Survival analysis is a collection of statistical analysis techniques that can be applied to situations in which the time to a given event, such as death, illness onset or recovery, is measured, but it is not necessary for all individuals to have reached this event during the overall time interval studied. The survival function, $S(t)$, is given by:

$$S(t) = P(t_s > t)$$

where
t = time
t_s = survival time

The survival function is also given by:

$$S(t) = 1 - (\text{cumulative distribution function of } t_s)$$

A survival curve is a plot of $S(t)$ (on the ordinate) versus t (on the abscissa). Instead of being drawn as continuous curves, sometimes survival curves are drawn in a stepwise fashion, with the steps occurring between estimated cumulative survival probabilities.

D True

The hazard function measures the likelihood of an individual experiencing a given event, such as death, illness onset or recovery, as a function of time.

E False

In a logistic regression model, the dependent variable or response variable is dichotomous or binary (e.g. yes/no or better/not better at the end of treatment) rather than continuous. The logistic regression model is used to predict the probability of this dependent variable on the basis of a set of independent variables, x_1 to x_n:

$$P(\text{event}) = 1/\{1 + \exp[-(\alpha_0 + \alpha_1 x_1 + \ldots + \alpha_n x_n)]\}$$

where the coefficients α_0 to α_n are estimated using a maximum likelihood method.

References/Further Reading

Revision Notes in Psychiatry, pp. 62, 67–8.

7 SOCIAL SCIENCES

Answers

7.1

A social class is a segment of the population sharing a broadly similar type and level of resources, with a broadly similar style of living and some shared perception of its common condition. The determinants of social class include

- education
- financial status
- occupation
- type of residence
- geographical area of residence
- leisure activities.

In British psychiatry, the following occupationally based classification given by the Office of Population Censuses and Surveys has traditionally been used

- social class I – professional, higher managerial, landowners
- social class II – intermediate
- social class III – skilled, manual, clerical
- social class IV – semi-skilled
- social class V – unskilled
- social class 0 – unemployed, students.

Members of the same household are assigned to the social class of the head of the household.

A True

B True

C False

They are classified as social class IV.

D False

They are classified as social class 0.

E True

References/Further Reading

Revision Notes in Psychiatry, p. 69.

7.2

A False

This is more likely to be diagnosed in the lower social classes.

B False

C False

This is more likely to be diagnosed in the lower social classes.

D True

E True

References/Further Reading

Revision Notes in Psychiatry, pp. 69–70.

7.3

The incidence and prevalence of many psychiatric disorders have been found to vary with social class. In particular, the following disorders are more likely to be diagnosed in lower social classes:

- schizophrenia
- alcohol dependence
- organic psychosis
- depressive episodes in women
- parasuicide/deliberate self-harm
- personality disorder.

The following disorders are more likely to be diagnosed in upper social classes:

- anorexia nervosa in women
- bulimia nervosa in women
- bipolar mood disorder.

A True

B True

C False

D True

E True

References/Further Reading

Revision Notes in Psychiatry, pp. 69–70.

7.4

Goldberg and Huxley (1980) described the existence of filters to psychiatric care, each of which depends on:

- social factors – such as age, sex, ethnic background, socioeconomic status
- service organization and provision, e.g. time and location of clinics, length of waiting list
- aspects of the disorder itself, e.g. its severity and chronicity.

These filters include:

- the decision to consult the general practitioner
- recognition of the disorder by the general practitioner
- the decision by the general practitioner as to whether or not to refer the patient to a specialist.

A True

B True

C True

D True

E True

References/Further Reading

Goldberg, D. and Huxley, P. (1980) *Mental Illness in the Community: the Pathways to Psychiatric Care.* London: Tavistock Publications.
Revision Notes in Psychiatry, p. 70.

7.5

In the model proposed by Parsons (1951) the social role of the doctor includes:

* defining illness
* legitimizing illness
* imposing an illness diagnosis if necessary
* offering appropriate help.

Doctors therefore control access to the sick role and they and patients have reciprocal obligations and rights.

The sick role was defined by Parsons (1951) as the role given by society to a sick individual, and was considered to carry rights or privileges and obligations. According to Parsons (1951), the sick role carries the following two rights for the sick individual:

* exemption from blame for the illness
* exemption from normal responsibilities while sick, such as the need to go to work.

The sick individual has the following obligations:

* the wish to recover as soon as possible, including seeking appropriate help from the doctor
* cooperation with medical investigations and acceptance of medical advice and treatment.

A False

Mechanic (1978) described illness behaviour, which is a set of stages describing the behaviour adopted by sick individuals. It describes the way in which individuals respond to somatic symptoms and signs and the conditions under which they come to view them as abnormal. Illness behaviour therefore involves the manner in which individuals:

* monitor their bodies
* define and interpret their symptoms and signs
* take remedial action
* utilize sources of help.

Illness behaviour includes the following stages:

* Initially well.
* Symptoms of the illness begin to be experienced.
* The opinion of immediate social contacts is sought.
* Contact is made with a doctor (or doctors).
* The illness is legitimized by the doctor(s).
* The individual adopts the sick role.
* On recovery (or death) the dependent stage of the sick role is given up.
* A rehabilitation stage is entered if the individual recovers.

The determinants of illness behaviour, according to Mechanic (1978), are

* the visibility, recognizability or perceptual salience of deviant signs and symptoms
* the extent to which symptoms are seen as being serious
* the extent to which symptoms disrupt the family, work and other social activities
* the frequency of appearance of deviant signs or symptoms, their persistence and the frequency of recurrence
* the tolerance threshold of exposed deviant signs and symptoms

- available information, knowledge and cultural understanding of exposed deviant signs and symptoms
- basic needs leading to denial
- the competition between needs and illness responses
- competing interpretations assigned to recognized symptoms
- the availability and physical proximity of treatment resources and the costs in terms of time, money, effort and stigma.

B True

C True

D True

E True

References/Further Reading

Mechanic, D. (1978) *Medical Sociology*, 2nd edn, Glencoe: Free Press.
Parsons, T. (1951) *The Social System*. Glencoe: Free Press.
Revision Notes in Psychiatry, pp. 71–2.

7.6

In assessing expressed emotion, the five relevant scales of the Camberwell Family Interview (CFI) are

- critical comments
- hostility
- emotional overinvolvement
- warmth
- positive remarks.

The first three of these are associated with high expressed emotion and predict relapse (Vaughn and Leff, 1976).

	Relapse rate in 9 months after discharge (%)
Antipsychotic medication, low expressed emotion family	12
Antipsychotic medication, high expressed emotion family, < 35 hours per week face-to-face contact	42
No antipsychotic medication, high expressed emotion family, > 35 hours per week face-to-face contact	92

A False

Although these constitute a scale of the Camberwell Family Interview, positive remarks, which express praise or approval of the patient, are not associated with high expressed emotion.

B False

The parents were held to communicate with the child (the future sufferer from schizophrenia) in abnormal ways, leading to feelings of ambivalence and ambiguity, with messages that were typically:

- vague
- ambiguous
- confusing.

Schizophrenia was said to develop as a result of exposure to such double-bind situations.

C True

These indicate unambiguous dislike or disapproval.

D False

This was held to be a cause of schizophrenia in which parental conflict, argument and hostility led to divided loyalties to mother and father on the part of the child (the future sufferer from schizophrenia).

E True

This entails exaggerated self-sacrificing or overprotective concern.

References/Further Reading

Revision Notes in Psychiatry, pp. 73–4.

Vaughn, C.E. and Leff, J.P. (1976) The influence of family and social factors on the course of schizophrenic illness. *British Journal of Psychiatry* **129**, 125–137.

7.7

A False

The concept of the schizophrenogenic mother was put forward by Fromm-Reichman in 1948. Schizophrenia was said to be a consequence of an inadequate relationship between the future sufferer from schizophrenia, as a child, and his or her mother. Characteristics of the schizophrenogenic mother were said to include her being:

* rejecting
* aloof
* overly protective
* overtly hostile.

B True

This concept was put forward by Bateson and colleagues in 1956.

C False

This concept was put forward by Lidz and colleagues in 1957. The parents were said to consist of a dominant and eccentric mother, and a passive and dependent father.

D True

This concept was put forward by Wynne and colleagues in 1958 and suggested that disordered communication took place between the parents of those with schizophrenia.

E False

In an outcome study of 200 patients, mainly with schizophrenia, Brown and colleagues in 1958 found that those discharged to their families had a poor outcome, with the highest relapse rate occurring in those families having close and frequent contact with the patients. Subsequent follow-up studies, such as those by Vaughn and Leff, have confirmed the association of high expressed emotion in families, characterized by the frequent, intense expression of emotion and a pushy and critical attitude by relatives to the patient, with an increased relapse rate in family members with schizophrenia.

References/Further Reading

Revision Notes in Psychiatry, pp. 73–4.

7.8

The following table gives some life-change values for life events in the Holmes and Rahe Social Readjustment Rating Scale:

Life event	Life-change value
Death of spouse	100
Divorce	73
Marital separation	65
Gaol term	63
Death of close family member	63
Personal injury or illness	53
Marriage	50
Being sacked from job	47
Retirement	45
Marital reconciliation	45
Pregnancy	40
Birth of child	39
Death of close friend	37
Child leaving home for good	29
Problems with in-laws	29
Problems with boss	23
Change in sleeping habits	16
Change in eating habits	15
Minor legal violation	11

The full Holmes and Rahe Social Readjustment Rating Scale introduced in 1967 consists of a self-report questionnaire containing 43 classes of life event.

A True

B False

The Life Events and Difficulties Schedule (LEDS) was devised by Brown and Harris and is a widely used instrument for current research into life events and psychiatric disorder. It has the following features:

- semistructured interview schedule
- 38 areas probed
- detailed narratives collected about events, including their circumstances
- high reliability
- high validity.

C False

In general the results of life event studies of mania are conflicting.

D True

There is strong evidence that threatening life events are more common before self-poisoning attempts (for example, Morgan *et al.*, 1975; Farmer and Creed, 1989).

E False

Death of one's spouse has a maximum life-change value of 100, as shown in the above table.

References/Further Reading

Farmer, R. and Creed, F. (1989) Life events and hostility in self-poisoning. *British Journal of Psychiatry* **154**, 390–95.

Morgan, H.G., Burns-Cox, C.J., Pocock, H. *et al.* (1975) Deliberate self-harm: clinical and socioeconomic characteristics of 368 patients. *British Journal of Psychiatry* **127**, 564–74.

Revision Notes in Psychiatry, pp. 76–7.

7.9

Many studies have found a relationship between life events and the onset of depression. In the 6–12 months before the onset, compared with normal controls, patients have a three to five times greater chance of having suffered at least one life event with major negative long-term implications (involving threat or loss). However, most people who experience adverse life events do not develop depression. Brown and Harris (1978) identified four vulnerability factors that make women more susceptible to suffer from depression following life events:

- loss of mother before the age of 11 years
- not working outside the home
- a lack of a confiding relationship
- having three or more children under the age of 15 years at home.

A False

This is one of the characteristics of the schizophrenogenic mother.

B True

C True

D False

This is one of the characteristics of the schizophrenogenic mother.

E False

This vulnerability factor entails having at least three children at home who are under the age of 15 years.

References/Further Reading

Brown, G.W. and Harris, T.O. (eds) (1978) *Social Origins of Depression: A Study of Psychiatric Disorder in Women*. London: Tavistock.
Revision Notes in Psychiatry, pp. 73, 76–7.

7.10

A total institution is an organization in which a large number of like-situated individuals, cut off from the wider social world for an appreciable period of time, together lead an enclosed formally administered round of life (Goffman, 1961). From his study of the large St. Elizabeth's Hospital, in Washington DC, USA, Goffman (1961) was one of the first to suggest that total institutions may be harmful.

A True

Other examples of total institutions include:

- prisons
- monasteries
- large ships.

B False

Political parties are examples of social institutions.

C False

The definition of a total institution is given above. It is a social institution that may be defined as an established and sanctioned form of relationship between social beings.

D True

E True

This is a concept introduced by Goffman.

References/Further Reading

Goffman, E. (1961) *Asylums: Essays on the Social Situation of Mental Patients and Other Inmates.* New York: Doubleday.
Revision Notes in Psychiatry, pp. 77–8.

7.11

All True.

According to Goffman (1961), patients were said to show various possible reactions to the mortification process, including:

- withdrawal
- open rebellion
- colonization – the patient pretends to show acceptance
- conversion
- institutionalization   actual acceptance both outwardly and inwardly.

References/Further Reading

Goffman, E. (1961) *Asylums: Essays on the Social Situation of Mental Patients and Other Inmates.* New York: Doubleday.
Revision Notes in Psychiatry, p. 78.

8.1

Abnormal movements that may occur in schizophrenia include:

- ambitendency
- echopraxia
- mannerisms
- negativism
- posturing
- stereotypies
- waxy flexibility.

A True

Here, the patient makes a series of tentative incomplete movements when expected to carry out a voluntary action.

B False

This is not a movement disorder. Dysprosody is a disorder of speech in which there is a loss of its normal melody.

C False

This is not a movement disorder. Schizophasia is a type of formal thought disorder, also called word salad or speech confusion, in which the speech is an incoherent and incomprehensible mixture of words and phrases.

D True

Negativism is a motiveless resistance to commands and to attempts to be moved.

E True

Echopraxia refers to the automatic imitation by the patient of another person's movements. It occurs even when the patient is asked not to do so.

References/Further Reading

Revision Notes in Psychiatry, pp. 84 and 85.

8.2

A False

There is a sudden interruption in the train of thought, before it is completed, leaving a 'blank'. After a period of silence, the patient cannot recall what he or she had been saying or had been thinking of saying.

B False

These are repeated regular fixed patterns of movement or speech that are not goal directed.

C True

This is a disorder of the form of speech in which thinking appears slow with the incorporation of unnecessary trivial details. The goal of thought is finally reached, however.

D False

These are repeated irregular movements involving a muscle group.

E True

These are repeated involuntary movements that appear to be goal directed.

References/Further Reading

Revision Notes in Psychiatry, pp. 84 and 85.

8.3

In perseveration (of both speech and movement), mental operations are continued beyond the point at which they are relevant.

A False

In this disorder of speech, the speech is fluent and rambling with the use of many words.

B False

This is a feature of formal thought disorder in which there is a disordered intermixture of the constituent parts of one complex thought.

C False

This is a disorder of the form of speech in which the answers to questions, although clearly incorrect, demonstrate that the questions are understood. For example, when asked 'What colour is grass?', the patient may reply 'Blue'.

D True

This is a type of perseveration of speech in which the patient repeats a word with increasing frequency.

E True

This is a type of perseveration of speech in which the patient repeats the last syllable of the last word.

References/Further Reading

Revision Notes in Psychiatry, p. 85.

8.4

All True.

Flight of ideas is a disorder of the form of speech in which the speech consists of a stream of accelerated thoughts with abrupt changes from topic to topic and no central direction. The connections between the thoughts may be based on:

- chance relationships
- clang associations
- distracting stimuli
- verbal associations – e.g. alliteration and assonance.

References/Further Reading

Revision Notes in Psychiatry, p. 85.

8.5

Schneider described the following features of formal thought disorder

* derailment
* drivelling
* fusion
* omission
* substitution.

A False

This is a disorder of self-awareness in which the surroundings do not seem real.

B False

This is a disorder of self-awareness in which one feels that one is altered or not real in some way.

C True

Heterogeneous elements of thought are interwoven with each other.

D True

A thought or part of a thought is senselessly omitted.

E True

A major thought is substituted by a subsidiary thought.

References/Further Reading

Revision Notes in Psychiatry, pp. 85–6, 90.

8.6

A delusion is a false belief based on incorrect inference about external reality that is firmly sustained despite what almost everyone else believes and despite what constitutes incontrovertible and obvious proof or evidence to the contrary. The belief is not one ordinarily accepted by other members of the person's culture or subculture (e.g. it is not an article of religious faith). When a false belief involves a value judgment, it is regarded as a delusion only when the judgment is so extreme as to defy credibility (DSM-IV).

A True

Othello syndrome is also known as

- delusional jealousy
- pathological jealousy
- delusion of infidelity.

It is a delusion that one's sexual partner is unfaithful.

B True

Also known as the delusion of doubles, l'illusion de sosies is a delusion that a person known to the patient has been replaced by a double. It is seen in Capgras' syndrome.

C True

This is a passivity phenomenon, i.e. a delusional belief that an external agency is controlling aspects of the self that are normally entirely under one's own control. Passivity phenomena include:

- thought alienation – the patient believes that his or her thoughts are under the control of an outside agency or that others are participating in his or her thinking; it includes
  - thought insertion – the delusion that certain of one's thoughts are not one's own, but rather are inserted into one's mind by an external agency
  - thought withdrawal – the delusion that one's thoughts are being removed from one's mind by an external agency
  - thought broadcasting – the delusion that one's thoughts are being broadcast out loud so that they can be perceived by others
- made feelings – the delusional belief that one's own free will has been removed and that an external agency is controlling one's feelings
- made impulses – the delusional belief that one's own free will has been removed and that an external agency is controlling one's impulses
- made actions – the delusional belief that one's own free will has been removed and that an external agency is controlling one's actions
- somatic passivity – the delusional belief that one is a passive recipient of somatic or bodily sensations from an external agency.

D False

Here similar thoughts are held to those in a delusion of reference, but with less than delusional intensity. (A delusion of reference is a delusion whose theme is that events, objects or other persons in one's immediate environment have a particular and unusual significance. These delusions are usually of a negative or pejorative nature, but also may be grandiose in content.)

E True

Erotomania is also known as de Clérambault's syndrome and is a delusion that another person, usually of higher status, is deeply in love with the individual.

References/Further Reading

Revision Notes in Psychiatry, pp. 88–9.

8.7

Sensory deceptions include

- illusions
- hallucinations
- pseudohallucinations.

Sensory distortions include

- hyperaesthesias
- hypoaesthesias
- changes in quality
- dysmegalopsia.

A False

This is a type of hyperaesthesia in which there is an increased sensitivity to sounds.

B False

This is a change in the quality of sensations of visual stimuli in which visual perceptions are coloured yellow.

C True

This is a type of hallucination, also known as a phantom mirror image, in which the patient sees himself or herself and knows that it is he or she.

D True

This is a type of hallucination in which moving objects are seen as a series of discrete discontinuous images.

E False

This is a type of dysmegalopsia (change in spatial form) in which objects are seen smaller or farther away than is actually the case.

References/Further Reading

Revision Notes in Psychiatry, pp. 89–90.

8.8

In receptive (sensory) aphasia (Wernicke's fluent aphasia), difficulty is experienced in comprehending the meaning of words. Types include:

- agnosic alexia
- pure word deafness
- visual asymbolia.

A False

Syntactical or central aphasia is a type of intermediate aphasia in which there is difficulty in arranging words in their proper sequence.

B True

In agnosic alexia, words can be seen but cannot be read.

C True

In pure word deafness, words that are heard cannot be comprehended.

D True

In visual asymbolia words can be transcribed but cannot be read.

E False

Nominal aphasia is a type of intermediate aphasia in which there is difficulty in naming objects.

References/Further Reading

Revision Notes in Psychiatry, p. 92.

9 PSYCHOANALYTIC THEORIES

Answers

9.1

In this model, it was held that the preconscious develops during childhood and serves to maintain repression and censorship. Its characteristic features include:

- outside awareness
- operating system – secondary process thinking
- motivating principle – the reality principle
- access – access can occur through focused attention
- system position
    - bound by time
    - word oriented
    - denotative
    - linear.

A False

Secondary process thinking is used.

B False

It is bound by time.

C True

D False

It is linear.

E False

It is outside awareness.

References/Further Reading

Revision Notes in Psychiatry, p. 95.

9.2

In this model, it was held that the unconscious contains memories, ideas and affects that are repressed. Its characteristic features include:

- outside awareness
- operating system – primary process thinking
- motivating principle – the pleasure principle
- access – access to its repressed contents is difficult, occurring when the censor gives way, for instance by becoming
  - relaxed
  - fooled
  - overpowered
- system position
  - no negation
  - timelessness (reference to time is bound up in unconsciousness)
  - image oriented
  - connotative
  - symbolic
  - non-linear.

A False

This is part of the system position of the conscious in this model.

B False

This is the motivating principle of the preconscious and conscious. (It is the pleasure principle that is the motivating principle of the unconscious.)

C True

D True

E True

References/Further Reading

Revision Notes in Psychiatry, pp. 95 and 96.

9.3

Attributes of primary process thinking include:

- displacement
- condensation
- symbolization.

Characteristics of primary process thinking include:

- timelessness
- disregard of reality of the conscious world
- psychical reality
- absence of contradiction
- absence of negation.

A False

B True

Symbols are used rather than words.

C True

All the meanings and several chains of association converge onto a single idea standing at their point of intersection.

D False

This is part of dream work and is the process of revising and/or elaborating the dream after awakening in order to make it more consistent with the rules of secondary process.

E True

An apparently insignificant idea is invested with all the psychical depth of meaning and intensity originally attributed to another idea.

References/Further Reading

Revision Notes in Psychiatry, pp. 96 and 97.

9.4

Freud referred to dreams as 'the Royal Road to the Unconscious'. Dreams were considered to be composed of:

- the day residue
- nocturnal stimuli
- unconscious wishes
- latent dream.

In turn, components of the latent dream include

- the day residue
- nocturnal stimuli
- unconscious wishes.

A True

These consist of both external stimuli, such as noise, moisture and touch, and internal stimuli, such as pain and urinary bladder distension.

B False

Secondary revision is also known as secondary elaboration and is the process of revising and/or elaborating the dream after awakening in order to make it more consistent with the rules of secondary process.

C True

This consists of memories of the waking hours before the dream that are particularly emotionally charged.

D False

This refers to the process whereby the latent dream is converted into the manifest dream. Operations that contribute to dream work can include

- displacement
- condensation
- symbolization
- secondary elaboration (secondary revision).

E True

References/Further Reading

Revision Notes in Psychiatry, p. 97.

9.5

Freud used the German word *trieb* to refer to a instinctual drive. Unfortunately, this has often been translated into the word 'instinct', a concept different from a 'drive'. Important instinctual drives identified by Freud were:

- libido
- eros
- thanatos.

A False

According to Sklar (1989):

> The transference is an unconscious process in which the patient transfers to the therapist feelings, emotions and attitudes that were experienced and/or desired in the patient's childhood, usually in relation to parents and siblings. It can be a passionate demand for love and hate in past relationships between the child and the adult. This is a complex field that includes the unconscious splitting of the therapist into masculine and feminine and locating unconscious affect and thinking of the 'child' part of the patient in relation to the maternal and paternal aspects of the therapist (i.e. Oedipal transference). Furthermore, the direction of such a transference can be both positive and negative. Thus, Freud encountered transference in many variations and certainly also in its hidden form, transformed by resistance. The therapist's transference represents on the one hand the most powerful ally but, on the other, in terms of transference's resistance, a therapeutic difficulty.

B True

This is the life preservation 'instinct'.

C False

The id is part of Freud's structural model of the mind. Most of the id is unconscious. It contains primordial energy reserves derived from instinctual drives. Its aim is to maximize pleasure by fulfilling these drives.

D True

This is the death 'instinct'.

E True

This is the sexual 'instinct' and energy of the eros.

References/Further Reading

Revision Notes in Psychiatry, pp. 97–9.
Sklar, J. (1989) Dynamic psychopathology. In: *Examination Notes for the MRCPsych Part I.* Puri, B.K. and Sklar, J., London: Butterworths/Heinemann.

9.6

The stages of psychosexual development identified by Freud were the:

- oral
- anal
- phallic
- latency
- genital.

A False

It typically takes place from around 3 years of age to around the end of the fifth year.

B False

Erotogenic pleasure is derived from sucking during the oral phase.

C True

Boys pass through the Oedipal complex. During the Oedipal phase of development they have an unconscious overly eroticized desire for their mother and wish to dispense with their competitive father who they fear may retaliate.

D True

Girls develop penis envy during the phallic phase of psychosexual development. It has been vigorously argued by many since the time of Sigmund Freud (for example the psychoanalyst Karen Horney) that this concept, with its implication that the psychology of women may depend on their feelings of genital inferiority and jealousy of men, is incorrect.

E True

Girls pass through the Electra complex. This is the female counterpart of the Oedipal complex in boys, with an unconscious overly eroticized desire for their father on the part of the girl, and a fear that this may lead to the loss of, or retaliation by, mother. These days this phase of development is usually referred to by psychoanalysts as the Oedipal phase in both boys and girls.

References/Further Reading

Revision Notes in Psychiatry, p. 99.

9.7

The archetypes of the objective psyche are energy-field configurations manifesting themselves as representational images having universal symbolic meaning and typical emotional and behavioural patterns. Five important types of archetype are identified in Jungian theory:

- anima
- animus
- persona
- shadow
- self.

A True

This is the masculine prototype within each person.

B False

Complexes surround archetypes and can be defined as feeling-toned ideas. They develop from an interaction of personal experiences and archetypal models.

C True

This represents repressed animal instincts arising from phylogenetic development and in dreams manifests itself as another person of the same sex.

D True

This is a central archetype holding together conscious and unconscious aspects, including future potential, archetypes and complexes.

E True

This is the outward mask covering the individual's personality and allowing social demands to be balanced with internal needs. Both a public and a private persona may be possessed by a person. The persona may be represented in terms of clothing in dreams.

References/Further Reading

Revision Notes in Psychiatry, p. 100.

9.8

Rather than explaining present events in terms of Freudian psychic determinism, Jungian theory employs:

* causality
* teleology
* synchronicity.

A True

This offers an explanation in terms of the future potential.

B False

This is an important concept in Freudian theory. Sklar (1989) described the important features of the countertransference in Freudian theory:

> The countertransference is the therapist's own feelings, emotions and attitudes to his patient. In the treatment mode, the therapist needs to screen out those that are mediated only by the therapist, and take note of those generated in the therapist from emotional contact with the patient. The latter can be an interesting aspect of the patient, e.g. the therapist may have the feelings of the patient as a child in relation to the patient enacting the parent. Thus, in the reverse transference, an aspect of the patient is located in the therapist *as a communication*.

C False

This is an important concept in Freudian theory. The superego in Freudian theory is concerned with issues of morality. It develops initially as a result of the imposition of parental restraint. Although more of the superego is conscious than is the case for the id, most of its activity occurs without consciousness.

D True

This offers an explanation in terms of causation at the boundary of the physical world with the psychical ('mystic') world.

E False

This is an important concept in Freudian theory, in which it is the motivating principle of primary process. The pleasure principle is mainly inborn. Pain/'unpleasure' is avoided and pleasure is sought through tension discharge. This leads to:

* wish fulfilment
* the discharge of instinctual drives.

References/Further Reading

Revision Notes in Psychiatry, pp. 96, 98 and 99.

Sklar, J. (1989) Dynamic psychopathology. In *Examination Notes for the MRCPsych Part I.* Puri, B.K. and Sklar, J., London: Butterworths/Heinemann.

9.9

Rejecting the critical importance of autoeroticism for the infant in Freudian theory, Klein believed instead that the paranoid position, later, under the influence of Fairburn, renamed the paranoid–schizoid position, developed as a result of frustration during the first year of life with pleasurable contact with objects such as the good breast. The paranoid–schizoid position, characterized by isolation and persecutory fears, developed as a result of the infant viewing the world as part objects, using the following defence mechanisms:

- introjection (internalization)
- projective identification
- splitting.

A True

In phantasy the subject transposes objects and their qualities from the external world into themselves.

B False

In this defence mechanism, excessive abstract thinking occurs in order to avoid conflicts or disturbing feelings.

C True

In this deficiency mechanism, 'good' objects, affects and memories are divided from 'bad'ones. It is often seen in patients with borderline personality disorder.

D True

In projective identification the subject not only sees the other as possessing aspects of the self that have been repressed, but constrains the other to take on those aspsects. It is a primitive form of projection.

E False

Here the external reality of an unwanted or unpleasant piece of information is denied.

References/Further Reading

Revision Notes In Psychiatry, pp. 101, 103 and 104.

9.10

Melanie Klein, who lacked any formal higher education and never developed a full theory of development, was a controversial figure in the British Psycho-Analytical Society. When she began developing her theories, Sigmund Freud viewed her as potentially challenging the work in child analysis of his daughter Anna Freud.

It is now known that Klein analysed her three children and wrote them up as disguised clinical cases. She proposed that the aim of child psychoanalysis was to 'cure' all children of their 'psychoses'.

A False

This concept is associated with Donald Winnicott. The transitional object is an object, which is neither oneself nor another person (including mother), that is selected by an infant between 4 and 18 months of age for self-soothing and anxiety reduction. Examples include a blanket or toy that helps the infant to go to sleep. It helps during the process of separation–individuation. In adults, transitional phenomena that may allow us to cope with loneliness and separation can include music, religion and scientific creativitiy.

B True

This is said to develop by the age of 6 months when the child no longer views the world in terms of part objects but realizes that objects are whole, and the world is not perfect.

C True

This is a phase of development that is held to occur during the first year.

D True

Like oral sadism, oral envy (of parental 'oral' sex) is held to occur during the first year. Together, oral envy and oral sadism lead to Oedipal impulses.

E True

This is said to occur in boys during early development.

References/Further Reading

Revision Notes in Psychiatry, pp. 101 and 102.

9.11

Donald Winnicott was a British paediatrician who became a psychoanalyst. He was a contemporary of Anna Freud and Melanie Klein, between whom he, at one time, tried to mediate. He made important contributions to object relations theory and his reputation has grown steadily since his death.

A True

Winnicott broadened the understanding of the countertransference from that of Freud, speaking of the objective countertransference. The objectivity derived from his belief that the countertransference was an understandable and normal reaction to the personality and behaviour of the analysand.

B True

The good-enough mother is a mother who responds to her baby's communications and meets his or her needs within an optimal zone of frustration and gratification.

C True

Good parenting by the mother, allowing her child to become increasingly autonomous while at the same time being dependent on her, results in the child being able to be himself or herself in the presence of his or her mother, and *vice versa*. This was termed the *capacity to be alone* in the presence of another.

D True

This is a play therapy technique.

E True

This is a therapeutic ambiance or setting that allows the patient to experience safety, and so facilitates psychotherapy.

References/Further Reading

Revision Notes in Psychiatry, p. 102.

Answers

10.1

During ontogeny, the midline neural tube differentiates into the following vesicles:

prosencephalon, which differentiates into the:

    telencephalon – gives rise to the cerebral hemispheres and contains the
        pallium
        rhinencephalon
        corpus striatum
        medullary centre

    diencephalon – consisting of the
        thalamus
        subthalamus
        hypothalamus

        epithalamus, consisting of the
            habenular nucleus
            pineal gland

mesencephalon, consisting of the:

    tectum, consisting of the corpora quadrigemina, made up of the
        superior colliculi
        inferior colliculi

    basis pedunculi
    tegmentum, containing

        the red nucleus
        fibre tracts
        grey matter surrounding the cerebral aqueduct

rhombencephalon, which differentiates into the:

    metencephalon – consisting of the
        pons
        oral part of the medulla oblongata
        cerebellum

    myelencephalon – the caudal part of the medulla oblongata

A True

B False

This is a diencephalic structure.

C False

The pons is derived from the metencephalon.

D True

E False

The superior colliculi are mesencephalic structures.

References/Further Reading

Revision Notes in Psychiatry, pp. 106–7.

10.2

On a morphological basis, neurones can be classified as:

- unipolar – the perikaryon has one neurite
- bipolar – the perikaryon has two neurites
- multipolar – each neurone has one axon and more than one dendrite.

    An alternative classification of neurones is on the basis of size

- Golgi type I – long axon
- Golgi type II – short axon terminating near the parent cell
- amacrine – no axon.

A False

B True

C False

This statement is true, but Schwann cells are not neurones. They are neuroglia. In addition to being part of myelinated peripheral nerves, Schwann cells encircle some unmyelinated peripheral nerve axons. Their functions include:

- peripheral nervous system myelin sheath formation
- neurilemma formation.

D False

E False

References/Further Reading

Revision Notes in Psychiatry, pp. 107 and 108.

10.3

The main types of neuroglia in the central nervous system are:

- astrocytes
- oligodendrocytes
- microglia
- ependyma.

A True

These are a type of ependymal cell. One of the functions of ependymal cells is to aid the flow of cerebrospinal fluid. Tanycytes line the floor of the third ventricle over the hypothalamic median eminence.

B False

Satellite cells are a type of neuroglia found in the peripheral nervous system. They are found in:

- sensory ganglia
- autonomic ganglia.

   Their functions include neuronal support in sensory and autonomic ganglia.

C True

These are a type of astrocyte. Astrocytes are multipolar and their functions include:

- structural support of neurones
- phagocytosis
- forming central nervous system neuroglial scar tissue
- contributing to the blood–brain barrier.

D True

Microglia are the smallest neuroglial cells and are most abundant in the grey matter. Their functions include acting as scavenger cells at sites of central nervous system injury.

E True

The functions of oligodendrocytes or oligodendroglia include:

- central nervous system myelin sheath formation
- phagocytosis.

References/Further Reading

Revision Notes in Psychiatry, pp. 107–8.

10.4

The core of the frontal operculum on the dominant side is Broca's area.

A False

B False

This is part of the superior mesial region of the frontal lobes.

C False

This is part of the superior mesial region of the frontal lobes.

D True

The frontal operculum consists of Brodmann areas 44, 45 and 47. These areas are named after Korbinian Brodmann who divided the cerebral cortex into 52 areas on histological grounds in the early twentieth century.

E True

Lesions in the non-dominant frontal operculum can lead to dysprosody.

References/Further Reading

Revision Notes in Psychiatry, p. 109.

10.5

The dorsolateral prefrontal cortex (DLPFC) contains Brodmann areas 8, 9, 10 and 46. Lesions in this region can lead to abnormalities in cognitive executive functions, impairment of verbal (left) or non-verbal (right) intellectual functions, memory impairments affecting recency and frequency judgements, poor organization, poor planning, poor abstraction and disturbances in motor programming. Left-sided lesions may cause impaired verbal fluency, while right lesions may cause impaired non-verbal (design) fluency.

A True

B False

This characteristically results from a lesion in Broca's area.

C True

D True

E True

References/Further Reading

Revision Notes in Psychiatry, p. 109.

10.6

The mesial temporal region consists of the

- parahippocampal gyrus (Brodmann areas 27 and 28)
- amygdala
- entorhinal cortex
- hippocampus.

Left-sided lesions can lead to anterograde amnesia affecting verbal information, while right-sided lesions can lead to anterograde amnesia affecting non-verbal information. Bilateral lesions can lead to verbal and non-verbal anterograde amnesia.

A False

The angular gyrus (Brodmann area 39) is part of the inferior parietal lobule.

B True

C True

D True

E False

The supramarginal gyrus (Brodmann area 40) is part of the inferior parietal lobule.

References/Further Reading

Revision Notes in Psychiatry, p. 110.

10.7

Lesions of the dorsal region of the occipital lobes (superior to the calcarine fissure) and adjoining parietal region (areas 7 and 39) can lead to partial (unilateral lesions) or a full-blown (bilateral lesions) Balint's syndrome, consisting of:

- simultanagnosia
- ocular apraxia or psychic gaze paralysis
- optic ataxia.

A True

B False

C True

D False

E False

The posterior part of the inferior parietal lobule together with the posterior part of the superior temporal gyrus (Wernicke's area) form the greater Wernicke's area. Left-sided temporoparietal junction lesions can lead to a receptive (sensory) aphasia (Wernicke's fluent aphasia), while right-sided temporoparietal junction lesions can lead to phonagnosia (impairment in the ability to recognize familiar voices) and amusia (impaired ability to recognize and process music).

References/Further Reading

Revision Notes in Psychiatry, pp. 110 and 111.

10.8

Authorities differ on the components of the basal ganglia. According to Snell (1987) the basal ganglia consist of the:

- corpus striatum
  - caudate nucleus
  - lentiform nucleus
- amygdala (amygdaloid nucleus)
- claustrum.

The lentiform nucleus consists of the:

- globus pallidus
- putamen.

A True

B True

C False

D True

E True

References/Further Reading

Revision Notes in Psychiatry, p. 111.

Snell, R.S. (1987) *Clinical Neuroanatomy for Medical Students*, 2nd edn. Boston: Little, Brown.

10.9

All true.

Efferents from the globus pallidus pass to the

- hypothalamus
- reticular formation
- substantia nigra
- subthalamus
- ventroanterior nucleus of the thalamus
- ventrolateral nucleus of the thalamus.

References/Further Reading

Revision Notes in Psychiatry, p. 112.

10.10

Alexander *et al.* (1986) have identified five parallel frontal–subcortical circuits that together form one of the main organizational networks of the brain and are central to brain–behaviour relationships. They connect specific regions of the frontal cortex with the basal ganglia and the thalamus in circuits that mediate:

* motor activity
* eye movements
* behaviour.

The overall structure of each circuit is as follows:

frontal lobe cortex → caudate nucleus → globus pallidus/substantia nigra → thalamus → frontal lobe cortex

The circuits are the:

* motor circuit
* oculomotor circuit
* dorsolateral prefrontal circuit
* lateral orbitofrontal circuit
* anterior cingulate circuit.

A True

This circuit originates in the supplementary motor area and subserves motor function.

B False

C True

This circuit originates in the frontal eye fields and subserves eye movements.

D False

E False

The *lateral* orbitofrontal circuit originates in the lateral orbital cortex and subserves personality.

References/Further Reading

Alexander, G.E., DeLong, M.R. and Strick, P.L. (1986) Parallel organisation of functionally segregated circuits linking basal ganglia and cortex. *Annual Review of Neuroscience* **9**, 357–381.
Revision Notes in Psychiatry, p. 112.

10.11

The limbic lobe was described by Broca in 1878 as an arrangement of cortical structures around the diencephalon, forming a border on the medial side of each cerebral hemisphere between the neocortex and the remainder of the brain. Cortical areas of the limbic lobe form the limbic cortex and include the:

- cingulate gyrus
- parahippocampal gyrus
- subcallosal gyrus.

Subcortical nuclei that are part of the limbic lobe include the:

- amygdaloid nucleus
- septal nucleus.

A True

B False
This is not a cortical area.

C False

D False

E True

References/Further Reading

Revision Notes in Psychiatry, p. 112.

10.12

Cortical areas that are generally considered to be part of the limbic system include the:

- cingulate gyrus
- gyrus fasciolaris
- hippocampal formation
  - dendate gyrus
  - hippocampus
  - parahippocampal gyrus
- indusium griseum
- olfactory tubercle
- paraterminal gyrus (precommissural septum)
- prepiriform cortex
- secondary olfactory area (entorhinal area)
- subcollosal gyrus
- subiculum.

A False

B True

C True

D False

E True

References/Further Reading

Revision Notes in Psychiatry, p. 113.

10.13

Subcortical nuclear groups that are generally considered to be part of the limbic system include the:

- amygdala (amygdaloid nucleus)
- anterior thalamic nucleus
- dorsal tegmental nucleus
- epithalamic nucleus
- habenula
- hypothalamic nuclei
- mammillary bodies
- raphe nucleus
- septal nucleus (septal area)
- superior central nucleus
- ventral tegmental area.

A True

B False

This nucleus is involved in the pathway of the optic nerve.

C False

This is one of the main motor nuclei of the oculomotor nerve.

D True

E False

This is one of the cerebellar nuclei. From medial to lateral in each cerebellar hemisphere, the cerebellar nuclei are as follows:

- fastigial
- globose
- emboliform
- dendate.

References/Further Reading

Revision Notes in Psychiatry, pp. 113 and 116.
Sciences Basic to Psychiatry, 2nd edn, p. 7.

10.14

Connecting pathways of the limbic system include the:

- anterior commissure
- cingulum
- dorsal longitudinal fasciculus
- fornix
- lateral longitudinal striae
- mammillotegmental tract
- mammillothalamic tract
- medial forebrain bundle
- medial longitudinal striae
- stria terminalis
- stria medullaris thalami.

A True

B True

C True

D False

This is a specific group of association fibres arranged in a curved shape running parallel to the cortical surface that, on the dominant (usually left) side, connects the more rostral Broca's area with Wernicke's area.

E True

References/Further Reading

Revision Notes in Psychiatry, pp. 113 and 116.

10.15

The corpus callosum is the largest set of interhemispheric connecting fibres. It lies inferior to the longitudinal fissure and superior to the diencephalon. It connects homologous neocortical areas. The main divisions of the corpus callosum (rostral first) are the:

- rostrum
- genu
- body
- splenium.

A True

B False

C False

The indusium griseum is a thin, vestigial layer of grey matter that covers the superior surface of the corpus callosum.

D False

E True

References/Further Reading

Revision Notes in Psychiatry, p. 115.

Snell, R.S. (1987) *Clinical Neuroanatomy for Medical Students,* 2nd edn. Boston: Little, Brown, pp. 275 and 277.

10.16

The Papez circuit is a concept introduced by Papez, in 1937, of a supposed limbic system reverberating circuit constituting the neuronal mechanism of emotion. It consisted of the:

- hippocampus
- hypothalamus
- anterior nucleus of the thalamus
- cingulate gyrus.

The postulated circuit was as follows:

      hippocampus → (via the fornix)

→   mammillary bodies of the hypothalamus → (via a synaptic connection)

→   anterior nucleus of the thalamus → (the neuroimpulse then radiates up)

→   cingulate gyrus → (via the cingulum)

→   hippocampus

A False

It is the anterior nucleus of the thalamus that was proposed to be part of the Papez circuit.

B True

C True

D False

This is part of the epithalamus and consists of a small group of neurones situated just medial to the posterior surface of the thalamus.

E True

References/Further Reading

Revision Notes in Psychiatry, pp. 115–16.

Snell, R.S. (1987) *Clinical Neuroanatomy for Medical Students,* 2nd edn. Boston: Little, Brown, p. 226

10.17

The oculomotor nerve has two motor nuclei:

- the main oculomotor nucleus (also known as the somatic efferent nucleus) – supplies all the extrinsic ocular muscles with the exception of the superior oblique and lateral rectus
- the accessory parasympathetic nucleus (also known as the Edinger–Westphal nucleus) – sends preganglionic parasympathetic fibres to the constrictor pupillae and ciliary muscles.

A True

B False

The superior oblique is supplied by the trochlear nerve.

C False

It is the abducent nerve that runs close to this bony structure. Raised intracranial pressure can cause the abducent nerve to be stretched over this structure. In addition, osteitis of the apex of the petrous temporal bone owing to otitis media can also damage it, leading to a unilateral palsy of this nerve. This is known as Gradenigo's syndrome.

D False

The oculomotor nerve is the third cranial nerve. The cranial nerves are

- I – olfactory
- II – optic
- III – oculomotor
- IV – trochlear
- V – trigeminal
- VI – abducent
- VII – facial
- VIII – vestibulocochlear
- IX – glossopharyngeal
- X – vagus
- XI – accessory
- XII – hypoglossal.

E True

Complete division of the oculomotor nerve leads to paralysis of the levator palpebrae superioris, and hence ptosis. Other features include:

- pupillary dilatation
- loss of the light and accommodation reflexes (owing to constrictor pupillae paralysis)
- divergent squint
- double vision.

References/Further Reading

Puri, B.K. and Sklar, J. (1990) *Revision for the MRCPsych Part I*. Edinburgh: Churchill Livingstone, p. 14.
Revision Notes in Psychiatry, pp. 116–120.

10.18

During embryogenesis, two groups of serotonergic neurones develop:

- a superior group – located at the boundary between the mesencephalon and the pons
- an inferior group – located from the pons caudally to the cervical spinal cord.

The superior group gives rise to the superior raphe nuclei and is largely responsible for the origin of ascending serotonergic fibres projecting to the forebrain. The main superior raphe nuclei are the:

- caudal linear nucleus (the most rostral)
- dorsal raphe nucleus
- median raphe nucleus
- supralemniscal nucleus.

Ascending fibres pass from the superior raphe nuclei, via pathways such as the dorsal raphe cortical tract (the largest pathway in primates) and the medial forebrain bundle (the largest pathway in the rat), to innervate the forebrain.

A True

B False

This is a hypothalamic nucleus that acts as a biological clock and possibly as the endogenous pacemaker for the nocturnal biosynthesis of melatonin from its precursor serotonin.

C True

D True

E False

The main noradrenergic nucleus in the central nervous system is the locus coeruleus, located in the dorsal pons.

References/Further Reading

Revision Notes in Psychiatry, pp. 122 and 123.
Sciences Basic to Psychiatry, 2nd edn, p. 69.

Answers

11.1

Macroscopic changes in Alzheimer's disease include:

- global brain atrophy
- ventricular enlargement
- sulcal widening.

    The atrophy is usually most marked in the frontal and temporal lobes.
    Macroscopic changes in Pick's disease include:

- selective asymmetrical atrophy of the anterior temporal lobes and frontal lobes
- knife-blade gyri
- ventricular enlargement.

A True

The atrophy tends to be more selective in Pick's disease, in which it affects the anterior temporal lobes and frontal lobes.

B False

Ventricular enlargement occurs in both Alzheimer's disease and Pick's disease.

C False

This is a feature of, for example, Parkinson's disease.

D False

Senile, or neuritic, plaques are a microscopic rather than a macroscopic feature.

E False

References/Further Reading

Revision Notes in Psychiatry, pp. 124 and 125.
Sciences Basic to Psychiatry, 2nd edn, pp. 225–6.

11.2

Histological changes in the cerebral cortex in Alzheimer's disease include:

- neuronal loss
- shrinking of dendritic branching
- reactive astrocytosis
- neurofibrillary tangles
- neuritic plaques (senile plaques).

There is a positive correlation between the number of neurofibrillary tangles and neuritic plaques, on the one hand, and, on the other, the degree of cognitive impairment. Histological changes seen commonly in the hippocampus include:

- granulovacuolar degeneration
- Hirano bodies
- neurofibrillary tangles
- neuritic plaques (senile plaques).

A True

Neurofibrillary degeneration leads to the formation of the highly insoluble neurofibrillary tangles that are made up of thick bundles of neurofibrils. They are stained well using silver impregnation. Ultrastructurally they are mainly composed of paired helical filaments of approximately 8 nm diameter with a periodicity of approximately 80 nm. Neurofibrillary tangles are occasionally present in the brains of elderly people. Their abundant presence in the brains of individuals with Alzheimer's disease, particularly in the cerebral cortex, is a characteristic neuropathological feature of this dementia. There is a correlation between their density and the degree of cognitive impairment in Alzheimer's disease.

B True

Electronmicroscopy reveals that each neuritic plaque contains an amyloid core made of A4 or beta amyloid. The numbers of neurofibrillary tangles and neuritic plaques correlate with the degree of cognitive impairment.

C True

Hirano bodies are intracytoplasmic neuronal inclusion bodies that are eosinophilic rod-shaped filamentous structures. They consist mainly of actin filaments.

D False

E True

In granulovacuolar degeneration there occur intracytoplasmic vacuoles of up to 5 mm in diameter that each contain an argyrophilic granule. This neuropathological change occurs mainly in the middle pyramidal layer of the hippocampus. Like neurofibrillary tangles, it is a neurodegenerative change that occurs in normal individuals with increasing age but is more prevalent in both Alzheimer's disease and progressive supranuclear palsy.

References/Further Reading

Revision Notes in Psychiatry, pp. 124–5
Sciences Basic to Psychiatry, 2nd edn, chapter 7.

11.3

Pick's bodies consist of:

- straight neurofilaments
- paired helical filaments
- endoplasmic reticulum.

A False

This is a feature of Lewy bodies.

B False

This is a feature of neuritic plaques.

C True

D True

E True

Histological changes in Pick's disease include:

- Pick's bodies
- neuronal loss
- reactive astrocytosis.

These changes may be seen in the:

- cerebral cortex
- basal ganglia
- locus coeruleus
- substantia nigra.

References/Further Reading

Revision Notes in Psychiatry, pp. 124, 125 and 126.

11.4

Lewy bodies contain:

- protein neurofilaments
- granular material
- dense core vesicles
- microtubule assembly protein
- ubiquitin
- tau protein.

A True

B False

This is a separate neuropathological feature.

C True

D True

E True

Compared with Parkinson's disease, in which Lewy bodies are also found, in dementia caused by Lewy body disease the density of Lewy bodies is much higher in the:

- cingulate gyrus
- parahippocampal gyrus
- temporal cortex.

References/Further Reading

Revision Notes in Psychiatry, pp. 125–6.

11.5

There may be little or no gross atrophy of the cerebral cortex evident in rapidly developing cases of Creutzfeldt–Jakob disease. In those surviving the longest, changes seen may include:

- selective cerebellar atrophy
- generalized cerebral atrophy
- ventricular enlargement.

Histological changes in the brain in dementia caused by Creutzfeldt–Jakob disease include:

- status spongiosus
- neuronal degeneration without inflammation
- astrocytic proliferation.

A True

B True

C False

This neuropathological change is seen in punch-drunk syndrome.

D False

This neuropathological change is seen in punch-drunk syndrome.

E True

A characteristic feature of the grey matter of the cerebral cortex in Creutzfeldt–Jakob disease is the presence of multiple vacuoles. This gives the cerebral cortex a spongy appearance, hence the name status spongiosus.

References/Further Reading

Revision Notes in Psychiatry, p. 126.
Sciences Basic to Psychiatry, 2nd edn, p. 216.

11.6

The main types of cerebral tumours, listed in order of relative frequency, are:

- gliomas
- metastases
- meningeal tumours
- pituitary adenomas
- neurilemmomas
- haemangioblastomas
- medulloblastomas.

Neurilemmomas are the commonest nerve sheath tumours and can affect the cranial nerves, particularly the eighth cranial nerve, the posterior nerve roots of the spinal cord and peripheral nerves. They are slow-growing and histologically are often cystic.

A False

Neurilemmomas are derived from Schwann cells. Haemangioblastomas are derived from blood vessels.

B True

Neurilemmomas are also known as Schwannomas because of the cells of origin.

C False

These are a type of glioma that are derived from ependymal cells.

D True

Neurilemmomas affecting the eighth cranial nerve, known as acoustic neuromas, are the commonest tumours to occur in the cerebello-pontine angle. They can give rise to:

- progressive deafness
- vertigo
- tinnitus.

As they increase in size, large tumours compress local structures and therefore also progressively give rise to:

- facial sensory loss (pressure on the ipsilateral fifth cranial nerve)
- masticatory weakness (pressure on the ipsilateral fifth cranial nerve)
- facial palsy (pressure on the ipsilateral seventh cranial nerve)
- lateral rectus palsy (pressure on the ipsilateral sixth cranial nerve)
- ipsilateral cerebellar signs
- features of brain stem compression.

E False

References/Further Reading

Revision Notes in Psychiatry, pp. 126–7.
Sciences Basic to Psychiatry, 2nd edn, p. 230.

11.7

A False

Bruton *et al.* (1990) found a significant reduction in the maximum anteroposterior length of formalin-fixed cerebral hemispheres in schizophrenia, compared with age- and sex-matched normal controls. Both hemispheres were shorter in schizophrenia compared with controls.

B False

Pakkenburg (1987) found that the volume of the white matter in post-mortem brains of patients with schizophrenia, compared with age- and sex-matched controls, did not differ significantly between the two groups.

C True

In the post-mortem brains of patients with schizophrenia, compared with age- and sex-matched controls, Pakkenburg (1987) found a significant reduction in the volumes of the:

* cerebral hemispheres
* cerebral cortex
* central grey matter.

D True

There is a slight but significant reduction in brain mass in schizophrenia, compared with controls, allowing for differences in height, body mass, sex and year of birth (Brown *et al.*, 1986; Pakkenburg, 1987; Bruton *et al.*, 1990).

E True

Ventricular enlargement has been found in a number of post-mortem studies of schizophrenic brains (e.g. Brown *et al.*, 1986; Pakkenburg, 1987; Bruton *et al.*, 1990). The ventricular enlargement particularly affects the temporal horn (Crow *et al.*, 1989), indicating temporal lobe neuropathology. Indeed, lateral ventricular enlargement is the most consistent structural neuroimaging finding in schizophrenia (Chua and McKenna, 1996).

References/Further Reading

Brown, R., Colter, N., Corsellis, J.A., *et al.* (1986) Postmortem evidence of structural brain changes in schizophrenia. Differences in brain weight, temporal horn area, and parahippocampal gyrus compared with affective disorder. *Archives of General Psychiatry* **43**, 36–42.

Bruton, C.J., Crow, T.J., Frith, C.D., Johnstone, E.C., Owens, D.G. and Roberts, G.W. (1990) Schizophrenia and the brain: a prospective clinico-neuropathological study. *Psychological Medicine* **20**, 285–304.

Chua, S.E. and McKenna, P.J. (1995) Schizophrenia – a brain disease? A critical review of structural and functional cerebral abnormality in the disorder. *British Journal of Psychiatry* **166**, 563–82.

Crow, T.J., Ball, J., Bloom, S.R., Brown, R., *et al.* (1989) Schizophrenia as an anomaly of development of cerebral asymmetry. A postmortem study and a proposal concerning the genetic basis of the disease. *Archives of General Psychiatry* **46**, 1145–50.

Pakkenberg, B. (1987) Postmortem study of chronic schizophrenic brains. *British Journal of Psychiatry* **151**, 744–52.

Revision Notes in Psychiatry, pp. 127–8.

11.8

Altshuler *et al.* (1990) studied the area and shape of the anterior hippocampus and parahippocampal gyrus in post-mortem brains from schizophrenic patients, non-schizophrenic suicide patients, and non-psychiatric controls. No significant differences were found in hippocampal area, but the parahippocampal gyrus was significantly smaller in the schizophrenic group compared with the control group.

Bogerts *et al.* (1990) also studied post-mortem brains of schizophrenic patients and control subjects. Compared with the controls, in the schizophrenic group the hippocampal formation was significantly smaller in the right and left hemispheres. The reduction in hippocampal volume in the male schizophrenics was greater than in the female schizophrenics.

A False

B True

The major of post-mortem studies have found a reduction in temporal lobe volume in schizophrenia. While the grey matter is reduced in volume, particularly at the level of the amygdala and anterior hippocampus, the volume of the white matter tends not to be reduced.

C True

Pyramidal cell disorientation in the hippocampus has been reported by Kovelman and Scheibel (1984) and by Conrad *et al.* (1991), although this failed to be found by Altshuler *et al.* (1987).

D False

Cytoarchitectural abnormalities have been reported in the entorhinal cortex in schizophrenia (Arnold *et al.*, 1991). These changes, which suggest disturbed development, included:

- aberrant invaginations of the surface
- disruption of cortical layers
- heterotopic displacement of neurons
- paucity of neurons in superficial layers.

Arnold *et al.* (1995) found that schizophrenic post-mortem brains had a smaller neurone size in the hippocampal regions of:

- the subiculum
- CA1
- layer II of the entorhinal cortex.

It is of note that the subiculum, CA1, and the entorhinal cortex are the major subfields of the hippocampal region that maintain the afferent and efferent connections of the hippocampus with widespread cortical and subcortical targets. It was therefore concluded that the smaller size of neurones in these subfields may reflect the presence of structural or functional impairments that disrupt these connections, which in turn could have behavioural sequelae.

E False

Almost all recent quantitative studies investigating the regions of greatest structural differences in schizophrenic patients have not shown significant gliosis. This negative finding is consistent with either of the following possibilities:

- the structural change in schizophrenic brains results from an embryonic insult before the third trimester (as the developing brain does not show reactive gliosis until approximately the third trimester)
- a neuropathological process occurs at or after the third trimester but does not usually initiate a glial reaction.

References/Further Reading

Altshuler, L.L., Casanova, M.F., Goldberg, T.E. and Kleinman, J.E. (1990) The hippocampus and parahippocampus in schizophrenia, suicide, and control brains. *Archives of General Psychiatry* **47**, 1029 34.

Altshuler, L.L., Conrad, A., Kovelman, J.A. and Scheibel, A. (1987) Hippocampal pyramidal cell orientation in schizophrenia. A controlled neurohistologic study of the Yakovlev collection. *Archives of General Psychiatry* **44**, 1094–98.

Arnold, S.E., Franz, B.R., Gur, R.C., Gur, R.E., *et al.* (1995) Smaller neuron size in schizophrenia in hippocampal subfields that mediate cortical–hippocampal interactions. *American Journal of Psychiatry* **152**, 738–48.

Arnold, S.E., Hyman, B.T., Van Hoesen, G.W. and Damasio, A.R. (1991) Some cytoarchitectural abnormalities of the entorhinal cortex in schizophrenia. *Archives of General Psychiatry* **48**, 625–632.

Bogerts, B., Falkai, P., Haupts, M., *et al.* (1990) Post-mortem volume measurements of limbic system and basal ganglia structures in chronic schizophrenics. Initial results from a new brain collection. *Schizophrenia Research* **3**, 295–301.

Conrad, A.J., Abebe, T., Austin, R., Forsythe, S. and Scheibel, A.B. (1991) Hippocampal pyramidal cell disarray in schizophrenia as a bilateral phenomenon. *Archives of General Psychiatry* **48**, 413–17.

Kovelman, J.A. and Scheibel, A.B. (1984) A neurohistological correlate of schizophrenia. *Biological Psychiatry* **19**, 1601–21.

Revision Notes in Psychiatry, pp. 128–9, 130.

11.9

A False

Idiopathic Parkinson's disease is characterized by a loss of dopaminergic neurones in the substantia nigra.

B False

Atrophy of the neostriatum is not a characteristic feature of tardive dyskinesia. Huntington's disease results from a mutation of the protein huntingtin and is characterized by a selective loss of discrete neuronal populations in the brain with progressive degeneration of efferent neurones of the neostriatum and sparing of dopaminergic afferents, resulting in progressive atrophy of the neostriatum.

C True

Macroscopic changes in idiopathic Parkinson's disease include:

*   depigmentation of the substantia nigra – particularly the zona compacta
*   depigmentation of the locus coeruleus.

D False

Both neuropathological and structural neuroimaging studies have indicated that hypoplastia of the cerebellar vermis as well as hypoplasia of the cerebellar hemispheres occurs in some subjects with autism. Ritvo *et al.* (1986) compared the cerebellums of four autistic subjects with those of three comparison subjects without central nervous system pathology and one with phenytoin toxicity. Total Purkinje cell counts were found to be significantly lower in the cerebellar hemisphere and vermis of each autistic subject than in the comparison subjects.

E True

Macroscopically, in Pick's disease there is selective asymmetrical atrophy of the frontal and temporal lobes, which, because of its severity, causes the gyri to become very thin – this being known as knife-blade atrophy of the gyri.

References/Further Reading

Revision Notes in Psychiatry, pp. 124–5, 130–2.

Ritvo, E.R., Freeman, B.J., Scheibel, A.B., *et al.* (1986) Lower Purkinje cell counts in the cerebella of four autistic subjects: initial findings of the UCLA-NSAC autopsy research report. *American Journal of Psychiatry* **143**, 862–6.

Answers

12.1

A True

High resolution structural images can be obtained using MRI (magnetic resonance imaging).

B True

This can be measured using ^{31}P MRS (31-phosphorus magnetic resonance spectroscopy). The ratio of the areas under the spectral peaks corresponding to phosphomonoesters and phosphodiesters enables a quantitative measure to be calculated of neuronal membrane phospholipid metabolism. This has been found to be abnormal in, for example, the prefrontal cortex in schizophrenia.

C True

This can be measured using ^{19}F MRS (19-fluorine magnetic resonance spectroscopy) with absolute quantitation. Such studies have been carried out in patients being treated with, for example, fluphenazine and fluoxetine.

D True

This can be measured using ^{7}Li-MRS (7-lithium magnetic resonance spectroscopy) with absolute quantitation.

E True

This can be measured using fMRI (functional magnetic resonance imaging).

References/Further Reading

Revision Notes in Psychiatry, p. 139.
Sciences Basic to Psychiatry, 2nd edn, p. 233.

12.2

Functional neuroimaging refers to techniques that, in contrast to anatomical images obtained using structural neuroimaging techniques, instead derive images reflecting types of information about the central nervous system such as:

- biochemical
- electrical
- physiological.

A False

B False

C True

D True

E True

References/Further Reading

Revision Notes in Psychiatry, pp. 137–9.

12.3

A False

B False

C False
31-Phosphorus is not radioactive.

D True
The basis of PET neuroimaging is as follows:

> a positron-emitting radioisotope or radiolabelled ligand is introduced into the cerebral circulation; routes commonly used are
> – intravenous administration (the radioactive substance is in solution)
> – by inhalation (the radioactive substance is in gaseous form)
→ blood flow ± cerebral tissue binding in the brain
→ emission of positrons
→ positron–electron interactions
→ dual γ photon emissions
→ detection of γ photons
→ computer reconstruction of emerging γ photon data
→ slice images of the distribution of the radioisotopes in the brain

The positron-emitting radioisotopes used can be produced in small cyclotrons.

E False

References/Further Reading

Revision Notes in Psychiatry, pp. 137–9.

12.4

Ionizing radiation, such as X-rays, beams of ionizing particles, such as electrons, and β and γ radiation, can cause direct damage to cellular DNA. It can also cause indirect damage to DNA by interacting with cellular water to give rise to potentially damaging free radicals.

A True

Patients are exposed to X-rays.

B False

C False

Proton magnetic resonance spectroscopy does not entail the exposure of patients to ionizing radiation.

D True

Patients are exposed to a positron-emitting radioisotope or radiolabelled ligand.

E True

Patients are exposed to a radioisotope or radiolabelled ligand.

References/Further Reading

Revision Notes in Psychiatry, pp. 137–9.

12.5

SPECT neuroimaging can give information about:

- regional cerebral blood flow (rCBF)
- ligand binding.

It is also of use in conditions in which the onset of the symptomatology being studied (e.g. epileptic seizures, auditory hallucinations) may occur at a time when the patient is not in or near a scanner; a suitable radioligand [e.g. technetium-99m hexamethylpropylene amine oxime (HMPAO)] can be administered at the material time and the patient scanned afterwards.

A True

B True

C False

This requires the use of structural neuroimaging techniques, for example MRI.

D False

This requires the use of serial structural imaging in conjunction with image registration.

E True

References/Further Reading

Revision Notes in Psychiatry, pp. 137–9.

Answers

13.1

In considering the origin of the membrane potential, the intracellular organic anions are unimportant because the membrane is relatively impermeable to them. The gradient between the extracellular and intracellular sodium ion concentrations is maintained by a powerful sodium pump that, in an active process involving ATP, pumps sodium ions out of the neurone against their concentration gradient in exchange for potassium ions entering the neurone. It is relatively difficult for sodium ions to enter the intracellular fluid, however, because of the impermeability of the resting neuronal membrane to them. Although potassium ions enter the neurone as a result of the action of the sodium pump, a continuous build-up of the intracellular potassium ion concentration is avoided because the neuronal membrane is relatively permeable to the potassium ion. In spite of this permeability potassium ions are prevented from equilibrating with respect to concentration because of their positive charge; the active extrusion of sodium ions leaves a negative intraneuronal electrical charge that both attracts the intracellular positively charged potassium ions and repels the extracellular negatively charged chloride ions.

A True

B False

The membrane potential, V_m, is defined as:

$$V_m = V_{in} - V_{out}$$

where V_{in} = the intracellular voltage or electrical potential and V_{out} = the extracellular voltage or electrical potential.

The resting membrane potential of a neurone is negative; for example that for a motoneurone is typically −70 mV.

C False

Energy for the process of maintaining the resting neuronal membrane potential is provided by ATP.

D False

E False

References/Further Reading

Revision Notes in Psychiatry, p. 140.
Sciences Basic to Psychiatry, 2nd edn, p. 37.

13.2

A False

It is in myelinated fibres that the action potential spreads by saltatory conduction. The action potential appears to jump from one node of Ranvier to the next, skipping the intervening myelinated parts.

B True

An action potential is propagated by the depolarization spreading laterally to adjacent parts of the neurone.

C True

The greater the diameter of the unmyelinated fibre the faster is the rate of transmission.

D True

The passage of an action potential along a neuronal axon is an all-or-none phenomenon. The initiating stimulus to a neurone is either sufficient to cause a degree of depolarization that increases the membrane potential beyond the critical threshold level (see part **E** below), in which case an action potential results, or else this threshold is not reached and there is no action potential. It is not possible for there to be a fraction of an action potential. Because the action potential is regenerated at each stage in its conduction along a neurone, it does not undergo any diminution with conduction. Therefore this is an exceedingly effective mode of transmission of nerve impulses over long distances.

E False

When a neurone is stimulated, the membrane potential at the point of stimulation becomes less negative; this is depolarization. If the degree of depolarization is greater than a critical threshold level then a nerve impulse or action potential is generated, during which the membrane potential rapidly becomes positive, and then negative again. The cause of the action potential is a change in the membrane permeability to sodium and potassium ions. As the membrane potential increases (i.e. becomes more positive) beyond the critical threshold level, there is a rapid increase in the membrane permeability to sodium ions that can be thought of as being caused by the opening up of membrane sodium ion channels. The rapid flow of sodium ions into the neurone continues until the membrane potential approaches the sodium ion equilibration potential, whereupon the sodium ion channels can be thought of as closing. At the same time the membrane permeability to potassium ions increases above the resting level and there is increased movement of (positively charged) potassium ions out of the neurone, thereby restoring the membrane potential to a negative value. When this part of the membrane is again at rest the original ionic concentration gradients are restored by means of the energy-consuming sodium pump.

References/Further Reading

Revision Notes in Psychiatry, pp. 140–1.
Sciences Basic to Psychiatry, 2nd edn, pp. 37–8.

13.3

Historically, it was observed that conduction usually occurred in one direction along a pathway of more than one neurone, in spite of the fact that one might expect a wave of excitation to be able to pass in either direction. The reason for this was found to be the fact that at the junction of two neurones, known as a synapse, there is no cytoplasmic continuity. Instead, there is a gap between the membrane of the presynaptic fibre and the membrane of the postsynaptic fibre. This gap is the synaptic cleft, and is often approximately 25 nm in width (one nanometre is 10^{-9} m).

A True

Synapses may be found between

- two neurones
- motoneurones and muscle cells
- sensory neurones and sensory receptors.

B False

There are two types of synapse:

- chemical – the commoner type, in which a chemical neurotransmitter is stored in presynaptic vesicles
- electrical – faster than chemical synapses, with direct membrane to membrane connection via gap junctions.

C False

Excitatory post-synaptic potentials, or EPSPs, occur in the post-synaptic membrane (because of depolarization) following release of an excitatory neurotransmitter from the presynaptic neurone at central excitatory synapses.

D False

Inhibitory post-synaptic potentials, or IPSPs, occur in the post-synaptic membrane (because of hyperpolarization) following release of an inhibitory neurotransmitter from the presynaptic neurone at central inhibitory synapses.

E True

One EPSP on its own is not usually sufficient to initiate an action potential. However, temporal and/or spatial summation may allow the degree of depolarization to reach the critical threshold. IPSPs, on summating with EPSPs, counter the effect of the latter.

References/Further Reading

Revision Notes in Psychiatry, p. 141.
Sciences Basic to Psychiatry, 2nd edn, pp. 39–40.

13.4

The anterior pituitary hormones include:

- corticotropin (adrenocorticotrophic hormone, ACTH)
- follicle-stimulating hormone (FSH)
- luteinizing hormone (LH)
- melanocyte-stimulating hormone (MSH)
- prolactin
- somatotropin (growth hormone, GH)
- thyrotropin (thyroid-stimulating hormone, TSH).

A True

B False

This is a posterior pituitary hormone.

C True

D False

This is secreted by the thyroid gland.

E False

This is a posterior pituitary hormone.

References/Further Reading

Revision Notes in Psychiatry, p. 142.

13.5

Hypothalamic release-inhibiting factors (hormones) include:

- MSH release inhibitory factor (MIH)
- prolactin release inhibitory factor (PIF) (dopamine)
- growth hormone release inhibitory factor (somatostatin).

   Hypothalamic releasing factors (hormones) include:

- corticotropin releasing factor (hormone) (CRF or CRH)
- gonadotropin releasing factor (hormone) (GnRF or GnRH)
- prolactin releasing factor (PRF)
- growth hormone releasing factor (hormone) (GRF or GRH; somatocrinin)
- thyrotropin releasing factor (hormone) (TRF or TRH).

A False

This is a hypothalamic releasing factor or hormone.

B False

This is growth hormone releasing factor.

C False

This is luteinizing hormone, an anterior pituitary hormone.

D True

E True

This is prolactin release inhibitory factor, hence the hyperprolactinaemia resulting from drugs with central antidopaminergic actions (such as typical antipsychotics).

References/Further Reading

Revision Notes in Psychiatry, p. 142.

13.6

The following stages normally occur during normal non-REM sleep:

- stage 0 – quiet wakefulness and shut eyes; EEG: alpha activity
- stage 1 – falling asleep; EEG: low amplitude, $\downarrow$ alpha activity, low-voltage theta activity
- stage 2 – light sleep; EEG: 2–7 Hz, occasional sleep spindles and K complexes
- stage 3 – deep sleep; $\uparrow$ delta activity (20–50%)
- stage 4 – deep sleep; $\uparrow\uparrow$ delta activity (> 50%).

A False

Alpha activity is a characteristic feature of the EEG during stage 0 sleep.

B True

C True

D False

E False

References/Further Reading

Revision Notes in Psychiatry, p. 143.

13.7

Features of REM sleep include:

- ↑ recall of dreaming if awoken during REM sleep
- ↑ complexity of dreams
- ↑ sympathetic activity
- transient runs of conjugate ocular movements
- maximal loss of muscle tone
- ↑ heart rate
- ↑ systolic blood pressure
- ↑ respiratory rate
- ↑ cerebral blood flow
- occasional myoclonic jerks
- penile erection or ↑ vaginal blood flow
- ↑ protein synthesis (rat brain).

A False

B False

C True

D False

E False

References/Further Reading

Revision Notes in Psychiatry, p. 143.

13.8

Features of non-REM sleep include:

- ↓ recall of dreaming if awoken during REM sleep
- ↓ complexity of dreams
- ↑ parasympathetic activity
- upward ocular deviation with few or no movements
- abolition of tendon reflexes
- ↓ heart rate
- ↓ systolic blood pressure
- ↓ respiratory rate
- ↓ cerebral blood flow
- penis not usually erect.

A True

B True

C False

In the monoaminergic model of the sleep–waking cycle:

- non-REM sleep is associated with serotonergic neuronal activity – raphe complex
- REM sleep is associated with noradrenergic neuronal activity – locus coeruleus

D False

REM sleep is also known as dreaming sleep. This is because sleep studies have consistently demonstrated that when a subject is woken while known from polysomnographic recordings to be in REM sleep, the subject is more likely to report that he or she is in the middle of a dream, than is the case when the subject is woken from non-REM sleep. However, dreaming is by no means confined to REM sleep. Therefore it is misleading to use the synonym dreaming sleep for REM sleep. What can be said with confidence is that a subject is more likely to remember that they were dreaming if woken during REM sleep. Non-REM sleep dreams are more likely to be simpler than REM dreams. For example, non-REM dreams may involve little or no movement in the dream scenes.

E True

References/Further Reading

Revision Notes in Psychiatry, p. 143.
Sciences Basic to Psychiatry, 2nd edn, p. 89.

13.9

In the cellular model of the sleep–waking cycle three groups of central neurones are of importance. These groups, and their corresponding neurotransmitters, are the:

• pontine gigantocellular tegmental fields (nucleus reticularis pontis caudalis) – acetylcholine
• dorsal raphe nuclei – serotonin
• locus coeruleus – noradrenaline.

According to this model, the gigantocellular tegmental field or 'on cells', which are inhibited by the dorsal raphe nuclei and the locus coeruleus (the 'off cells'), are responsible for causing the onset of REM sleep, during which a gradual increase in the activity of the off cells leads to an inhibition of the on cells and the restoration of non-REM sleep or wakefulness. Evidence in support of this model includes the finding that the injection of very small quantities of cholinergic agents into the gigantocellular tegmental field leads rapidly to the onset of REM sleep. On the other hand, ablation experiments have failed to lend support to this model.

A False

The neurotransmitter is dopamine.

B False

C True

D True

E False

References/Further Reading

Revision Notes in Psychiatry, p. 143.
Sciences Basic to Psychiatry, 2nd edn, pp. 91–2.

13.10

Normal EEG rhythms are classified according to frequency as follows:

- delta – frequency < 4 Hz
- theta – 4 Hz ≤ frequency < 8 Hz
- alpha – 8 Hz ≤ frequency < 13 Hz
- beta – frequency ≥ 13 Hz.

A False

This frequency is classed as a delta rhythm.

B False

This frequency is classed as an alpha rhythm.

C True

D True

E False

This frequency is classed as an alpha rhythm.

References/Further Reading

Revision Notes in Psychiatry, p. 144.

13.11

A False

Mu activity occurs over the motor cortex.

B False

Mu activity is related to motor activity and is abolished by movement of the contralateral limb.

C False

Lambda activity occurs over the occipital region in subjects with their eyes open.

D True

Lambda activity is related to ocular movements during visual attention.

E False

References/Further Reading

Revision Notes in Psychiatry, p. 144.

13.12

A False

The positions of the electrodes is usually according to the International 10-20 (not 10-30) System, which entails measurements from the following scalp landmarks:

- the nasion
- the inion
- the right auricular depression
- the left auricular depression.

In this system, proportions of scalp distances are 10% or 20%, and mid-line electrodes are denoted by the subscript z.

B True

Spikes are transient high peaks that last less than 80 ms.

C True

This is a specialized recording technique in which sphenoidal electrodes are inserted between the mandibular coronoid notch and the zygoma. They can be used to obtain recordings from the inferior temporal lobe.

D False

Sharp waves are conspicuous sharply defined wave formations that rise rapidly, fall more slowly and last more than 80 ms.

E True

This is a specialized recording technique in which electrodes are positioned in the superior part of the nasopharynx. Nasopharyngeal leads can be used to obtain recordings from the inferior and medial temporal lobe.

References/Further Reading

Revision Notes in Psychiatry, p. 144.

13.13

A False

Amitriptyline causes an increase in delta activity.

B False

This is not a characteristic feature of lithium at therapeutic levels. Therapeutic levels of lithium lead to only small EEG effects that are likely to be missed on visual analysis of routine recordings.

C False

In general, the action of antipsychotics, such as chlorpromazine, on beta activity is to decrease it.

D False

Benzodiazepines cause an increase in beta activity.

E False

Barbiturates do not increase such activity.

References/Further Reading

Revision Notes in Psychiatry, pp. 144–5.

14 NEUROCHEMISTRY

Answers

14.1

A False

The major carboxylterminal amidated cholecystokinin peptide in the brain is CCK 8. In the gastrointestinal tract, the larger forms that are more abundant than CCK 8 are:

- CCK 22
- CCK 33
- CCK 39
- CCK 58.

Cholecystokinin is located in high concentrations in the mammalian central nervous system, particularly in the cerebral cortex, hypothalamus and parts of the limbic system. Cholecystokinin has been found in mammalian studies to coexist with classical neurotransmitters. For example, cholecystokinin coexists with dopamine in the mesencephalon, with GABA in the cerebral cortex and with 5-hydroxytryptamine in the medulla oblongata.

B True

Galanin is a neuropeptide that coexists with the following neurotransmitters in parts of the brain:

- GABA
- 5-HT
- noradrenaline
- NPY (neuropeptide Y).

It mainly has an inhibitory neurotransmitter action on the secretion of other neurotransmitters and hormones, via G_1 protein-coupled receptors and ion channels.

C False

Proopiomelanocortin (POMC) is an opioid peptide precursor from which is derived the following peptides:

- corticotropin
- β-lipotropin
- γ-lipotropin
- CLIP (corticotropin-like immunoreactive peptide)
- α-endorphin
- β-endorphin
- γ-endorphin
- α-MSH
- β-MSH
- γ-MSH
- met-enkephalin.

The major central nervous system site that the POMC gene is expressed in is the pituitary gland.

D True

Acetylcholine (ACh) is a classical neurotransmitter.

E True

Nitric oxide (NO) is a second messenger and neurotransmitter. It is normally produced from reactions catalyzed by the Ca^{2+}-dependent enzyme nitric oxide synthase (NOS) in which the precursor amino acid arginine is converted into citrulline.

References/Further Reading

Revision Notes in Psychiatry, p. 152.
Sciences Basic to Psychiatry, 2nd edn, chapters 2 and 3.

14.2

There is now strong evidence that endogenous opioid peptides, such as the dynorphins, act as neurotransmitters.

A True

Corticotropin (ACTH) is a POMC-derived peptide (see the answer to the previous question).

B True

This is a proenkephalin-derived peptide.

C False

Glycine is an inhibitory amino acid neurotransmitter. (As it consists of only one amino acid, it is not a peptide.)

D False

Dopamine is not a peptide.

E True

This is a prodynorphin-derived peptide.

References/Further Reading

Revision Notes in Psychiatry, p. 152.
Sciences Basic to Psychiatry, 2nd edn, chapters 2 and 3.

14.3

Transmitter release from synaptic vesicles takes place by exocytosis in a process controlled by Ca^{2+} influx. The Ca^{2+} enters via voltage-dependent ion channels. Importantly, Na^+ influx and/or K^+ efflux are not needed for transmitter release.

A False

B False

C True

As the number of vesicles released is an integer, transmitter release is essentially quantal in nature.

D True

E True

References/Further Reading

Revision Notes in Psychiatry, p. 146.

14.4

All true.

Ca^{2+} influences or regulates:

- the probability of vesicular transmitter release
- vesicular fusion
- the transport of synaptic vesicles to the presynaptic active zone of exocytosis
- post-tetanic potentiation
- tonic depolarization of the presynaptic neurone.

References/Further Reading

Revision Notes in Psychiatry, p. 146.

14.5

The types of glutamate receptor recognized are:

- NMDA (*N*-methyl-D-aspartate) receptors
- AMPA (α-amino-3-hydroxy-5-methyl-4-isoxazole propionic acid) receptors
- KA (kainic acid) receptors
- mGluRs (metabotropic glutamate receptors) (= *trans*-ACPD receptors).

The first three classes are ionotropic glutamate receptors that are coupled directly to cation-specific ion channels.

A True

KA receptors include:

- GluR5
- GluR6
- GluR7
- KA1
- KA2.

B False

M2 are muscarinic cholinergic receptors.

C True

The mGluRs are coupled to G proteins, unlike the other classes of glutamate receptor. At the time of writing, the following subtypes have been cloned:

- mGluR1
- mGluR2
- mGluR3
- mGluR4
- mGluR5
- mGluR6.

These have been categorized into the following subgroups:

- subgroup I = mGluR1 and mGluR5
- subgroup II = mGluR2 and mGluR3
- subgroup III = mGluR4 and mGluR6.

The effector system for subgroup I involves stimulation of phospholipase C, while that for both subgroup II and subgroup III involves inhibition of adenylate cyclase.

D True

At the time of writing the NMDA receptor subtype is believed to include two families of subunits:

- NMDAR1 (= NR1)
- NMDAR2 (= NR2).

Variants of NMDAR2 are modulatory subunits that form heteromeric channels but not homomeric channels.

E True

AMPA receptors can be formed from one or any two of:

- GluR1
- GluR2
- GluR3
- GluR4.

References/Further Reading

Revision Notes in Psychiatry, pp. 148–9.
Sciences Basic to Psychiatry, 2nd edn, chapter 3.

14.6

The primary biosynthetic pathway is:

      tyrosine
→   DOPA
→   dopamine
→   noradrenaline

A False

B False

This is the enzyme catechol-*O*-methyltransferase that may begin the metabolic degradation of noradrenaline.

C True

D False

MHPG (3-methoxy-4-hydroxyphenylglycol) is a metabolic breakdown product from noradrenaline.

E True

Tyrosine is converted to DOPA (3,4-dihydroxyphenylalanine) via the action of the enzyme tyrosine hydroxylase.

References/Further Reading

Revision Notes in Psychiatry, pp. 149–50.

14.7

The metabolic degradation of noradrenaline may begin with the action of either catechol-*O*-methyltransferase (COMT) or monoamine oxidase (MAO). The catabolic pathway starting with the action of COMT is as follows:

    noradrenaline
→   normetanephrine
→   3-methoxy-4-hydroxyphenylglycolaldehyde
→   VMA (vanillyl mandelic acid)

A True

3-methoxy-4-hydroxymandelic acid is VMA.

B False

The catabolic pathway of noradrenaline starting with the action of MAO has two major branches. The first branch is as follows:

    noradrenaline
→   3,4-dihydroxyphenylglycolaldehyde
→   3,4-dihydroxymandelic acid
→   VMA (vanillyl mandelic acid)

   The second branch is as follows:

    noradrenaline
→   3,4-dihydroxyphenylglycolaldehyde
→   3,4-dihydroxyphenylglycol
→   MHPG

C False

DOPAC is dihydroxyphenylacetic acid and is produced in the catabolic pathway that starts with the action of MAO on dopamine.

D True

E False

This is homovanillic acid.

References/Further Reading

Revision Notes in Psychiatry, pp. 150 and 151.

14.8

The primary biosynthetic pathway of serotonin (5-HT) is:

> tryptophan
> $\rightarrow$ 5-hydroxytryptophan
> $\rightarrow$ serotonin

The corresponding enzymes are:

- tryptophan hydroxylase (acts on tryptophan)
- 5-hydroxytryptophan decarboxylase = amino acid decarboxylase (acts on 5-hydroxytryptophan).

A True

B False

5-HIAA (5-hydroxyindoleacetic acid) is the main metabolic breakdown product from serotonin.

C True

D False

MAO_A (MAO type A) is the enzyme that catalyses the following metabolic degradation of serotonin:

> serotonin
> $\rightarrow$ 5-HIAA

E False

References/Further Reading

Revision Notes in Psychiatry, pp. 150–151.

14.9

The catabolic pathway of dopamine starting with the action of MAO is as follows:
dopamine

$\rightarrow$ 3,4-dihydroxyphenylacetaldehyde
$\rightarrow$ DOPAC (dihydroxyphenylacetic acid)
$\rightarrow$ HVA

The corresponding enzymes are:

* MAO (acts on dopamine)
* aldehyde dehydrogenase (acts on 3,4-dihydroxyphenylacetaldehyde)
* COMT (acts on DOPAC).

A False

DOPA is in the primary anabolic biosynthetic pathway to dopamine:

tyrosine
$\rightarrow$ DOPA (3,4-dihydroxyphenylalanine)
$\rightarrow$ dopamine.

B True

C True

D True

E True

This is HVA.

References/Further Reading

Revision Notes in Psychiatry, p. 151.

14.10

A False

GABA is derived from glutamic acid via the action of GAD (glutamic acid decarboxylase).

B False

The GABA receptor superfamilies may be large, with multiple types of GABA subunits having been cloned. In general, there are two main types of receptor, the main effects of which are:

$GABA_A \rightarrow \uparrow Cl^-$ (via a receptor-gated ion channel)

$GABA_B \rightarrow \uparrow K^+ \pm Ca^{2+}$ effects (via G protein coupling)

C False

D True

E True

The metabolic breakdown of GABA to glutamic acid and succinic semialdehyde involves the action of GABA transaminase (GABA-T).

References/Further Reading

Revision Notes in Psychiatry, pp. 148 and 152.

14.11

A True

Cholinergic receptors transduce signals via coupling with G proteins. At the time of writing, the following types are recognized:

- nicotinic
- M1 (muscarinic)
- M2 (muscarinic)
- M3 (muscarinic)
- M4 (muscarinic)
- M5 (muscarinic).

B True

Acetylcholine is derived from acetyl CoA and choline, in a reaction catalysed by choline acetyltransferase.

C False

D False

After release into the synaptic cleft, acetylcholine is hydrolysed by cholinesterase into choline and ethanoic (acetic) acid.

E True

References/Further Reading

Revision Notes in Psychiatry, pp. 148 and 152.

15 GENERAL PRINCIPLES OF PSYCHOPHARMACOLOGY

Answers

15.1

A True

Chlorpromazine was synthesized by Charpentier, who was attempting to create an antihistaminergic agent for anaesthetic use.

B False

Haloperidol was synthesized by Janssen.

C False

Lithium is an element and therefore was not synthesized by humans.

D False

Following its synthesis by Charpentier, Laborit reported that chlorpromazine could induce an artificial hibernation.

E True

The benzodiazepine chlordiazepoxide was synthesized by Sternbach (working for Roche).

References/Further Reading

Revision Notes in Psychiatry, pp. 153–4.

15.2

A True

The clinical use of MAOIs in psychiatry arose from the observation of elevated mood in patients with tuberculosis being treated with the MAOI iproniazid. Less toxic MAOIs were subsequently developed. Kline was one of the first to report the value of MAOI treatment in depression.

B True

Kuhn observed the antidepressant action of imipramine while studying chlorpromazine-like agents.

C True

Following his finding from animal experiments that lithium caused lethargy, Cade observed that it led to clinical improvement in a patient with mania. In turn this led to the clinical introduction of lithium in psychiatry.

D True

The efficacy of chlorpromazine in the treatment of psychosis was reported by Paraire and Sigwald, and by Delay and Deniker.

E True

Kane and colleagues reported positive results from their multicentre double-blind study of clozapine versus chlorpromazine in treatment-resistant schizophrenia. Subsequent studies showed that social functioning also improved in response to clozapine.

References/Further Reading

Revision Notes in Psychiatry, pp. 153–4.

15.3

A False

Tricyclic antidepressants and monoamine oxidase inhibitors (MAOIs) were introduced between 1955 and 1958.

B False

The selective serotonin re-uptake inhibitors (SSRIs) were introduced in the 1980s.

C True

In 1886 Lange proposed the use of lithium for treating excited states. Lithium was introduced into clinical psychiatric use by Cade in 1949. Following his finding from animal experiments that lithium caused lethargy, Cade observed (in 1948) that it led to clinical improvement in a patient with mania.

D True

Important dates in the introduction of typical antipsychotics in psychiatric treatment in the twentieth century include:

- 1950 – chlorpromazine synthesized by Charpentier, who was attempting to synthesize an antihistaminergic agent for anaesthetic use; Laborit then reported that chlorpromazine could induce an artificial hibernation
- the efficacy of chlorpromazine in the treatment of psychosis was reported by Paraire and Sigwald in 1951, and by Delay and Deniker in 1952
- 1958 – haloperidol was synthesized by Janssen.

E False

The first barbiturate, barbituric acid (malonylurea), was synthesized in 1864. The barbiturates were introduced in 1903.

References/Further Reading

Revision Notes in Psychiatry, pp. 153–4.

15.4

The following is a guide to the classification of some typical antipsychotics:

- phenothiazines: aliphatic
  - chlorpromazine
  - methotrimeprazine
  - promazine
- phenothiazines: piperazines
  - fluphenazine
  - trifluoperazine
  - perphenazine
  - prochlorperazine
- phenothiazines: piperidines
  - pipothiazine palmitate
  - pericyazine
- butyrophenones
  - haloperidol
  - droperidol
  - benperidol
  - trifluperidol
- thioxanthenes
  - flupenthixol
  - zuclopenthixol
- diphenylbutylpiperidines
  - pimozide
  - fluspirilene.

A False

Perphenazine is a member of the piperazine group of phenothiazines.

B False

Procyclidine is not an antipsychotic.

C True

D False

Thioridazine is a member of the piperidine group of phenothiazines.

E True

References/Further Reading

Revision Notes in Psychiatry, pp. 154–5.

15.5

Antimuscarinic (anticholinergic) drugs used in the treatment of parkinsonism resulting from pharmacotherapy with antipsychotics include:

- procyclidine
- benzhexol
- benztropine
- orphenadrine
- biperiden
- methixene.

A False

This is an atypical antipsychotic.

B True

C True

D True

E False

This is a typical antipsychotic.

References/Further Reading

Revision Notes in Psychiatry, pp. 154–5.

15.6

Monoamine oxidase inhibitors (MAOIs) include:

- hydrazine compounds
    - phenelzine
    - isocarboxazid
- non-hydrazine compounds
    - tranylcypromine.

A True

B False

This is a tetracyclic antidepressant.

C False

This is a relatively new antidepressant that inhibits serotonin re-uptake and also selectively blocks serotonin receptors.

D True

E True

This is an antidepressant that acts by being a reversible inhibitor of monoamine oxidase type A (MAO_A).

References/Further Reading

Revision Notes in Psychiatry, p. 156.

16 PHARMACOKINETICS

Answers

16.1

Parenteral administration includes administration via the following routes:

* intramuscular
* intravenous
* subcutaneous
* inhalational
* topical.

In contrast, enteral administration routes use the gastrointestinal tract, from which the drug is absorbed into the circulation. They include administration via the following routes:

* oral
* buccal
* sublingual
* rectal.

A False

B False

C True

D True

E True

References/Further Reading

Revision Notes in Psychiatry, p. 160.

16.2

The rate of absorption of drugs administered intramuscularly is increased in the following circumstances:

- lipid-soluble drugs
- drugs with a low relative molecular mass
- ↑ muscle blood flow – e.g. after physical exercise or during emotional excitement.

A True

B False

C True

D False

There is reduced muscle blood flow in cardiac failure.

E True

References/Further Reading

Revision Notes in Psychiatry, p. 161.

16.3

The volume of distribution is a theoretical concept relating the mass of a drug in the body to the blood or plasma concentration:

> volume of distribution = (mass of a drug in the body at a given time) ÷ (the concentration of the drug at that time in the blood or the plasma).

A True

Increased lipid solubility, as is the case for most psychotropic drugs, is associated with an increased volume of distribution.

B True

An increase in body mass is usually associated with an increase in adipose tissue, which in turn leads to an increase in the volume of distribution.

C False

Increasing age is associated with a reduction in the proportion of lean tissue in the body, which in turn leads to an increased volume of distribution.

D False

A higher volume of distribution in general corresponds to a shorter duration of drug action.

E False

In general the volume of distribution tends to be lower for drugs that are highly protein bound.

References/Further Reading

Revision Notes in Psychiatry, pp. 162–3.
Sciences Basic to Psychiatry, 2nd edn, pp. 137–8.

16.4

Drugs circulate around the body partly bound to plasma proteins and partly free in the water phase of plasma. The extent of plasma protein binding varies with a number of factors:

- plasma drug concentration
- plasma protein concentration – ↓ in
  - hepatic disease
  - renal disease
  - cardiac failure
  - malnutrition
  - carcinoma
  - surgery
  - burns
- drug interactions
  - displacement
  - plasma protein tertiary structure change
- concentration of physiological substances – e.g. urea, bilirubin and free fatty acid.

A False

Plasma protein binding is reversible and competitive and acts as a reservoir for the drug.

B False

The main plasma binding protein for acidic drugs is albumin, while basic drugs, including many psychotropic drugs, can also bind to other plasma proteins, such as lipoprotein and α_1-acid glycoprotein.

C False

D True

E True

References/Further Reading

Revision Notes in Psychiatry, pp. 162–3.

16.5

A True

Components of the blood–brain barrier include:

- tight junctions between adjacent cerebral capillary endothelial cells
- cerebral capillary basement membrane
- gliovascular membrane.

B False

C False

A high rate of penetration of the blood–brain barrier occurs for non-polar highly lipid soluble drugs because the brain is a highly lipid organ. Most psychotropic drugs, being highly lipid soluble, can therefore easily cross the blood–brain barrier.

D True

Some small molecules and ions diffuse readily into the brain and cerebrospinal fluid from the cerebral circulation, e.g. lithium ions.

E False

Active transport mechanisms are used to cross the blood–brain barrier by some physiological substances and drugs, e.g. levodopa.

References/Further Reading

Revision Notes in Psychiatry, p. 163.

16.6

Hepatic phase I biotransformation leads to a change in the drug molecular structure by the following non-synthetic reactions:

- oxidation – the most common
- hydrolysis
- reduction.

The most important type of oxidation reaction is that carried out by microsomal mixed-function oxidases, involving the cytochrome P450 isoenzymes.

A True

B False

Lithium ions cannot be metabolized.

C True

D False

Hepatic phase II biotransformation is a synthetic reaction involving conjugation between a parent drug/drug metabolite/endogenous substance and a polar endogenous molecule/group. Examples of the latter include:

- glucuronic acid
- sulphate
- acetate
- glutathione
- glycine
- glutamine.

The resulting water-soluble conjugate can be excreted by the kidney if the relative molecular mass is less than approximately 300. If the relative molecular mass is greater than approximately 300, the conjugate can be excreted in the bile.

E True

The first-pass effect (first-pass metabolism or presystemic elimination) is the metabolism undergone by an orally absorbed drug during its passage from the hepatic portal system through the liver before entering the systemic circulation. It varies between individuals and may be reduced by, for example, hepatic disease, food or drugs that increase hepatic blood flow.

References/Further Reading

Revision Notes in Psychiatry, p. 164.

Answers

17.1

All true.

The atypical antipsychotics have a greater action than do typical antipsychotics on receptors other than dopamine D2 receptors. Clozapine, the archetypal atypical antipsychotic, has a higher potency of action than do typical antipsychotics on the following receptors:

- 5-HT_2
- D4
- D1
- muscarinic
- α-adrenergic.

References/Further Reading

Revision Notes in Psychiatry, p. 167.

17.2

In general, typical antipsychotics such as chlorpromazine are postulated to act clinically by causing postsynaptic blockade of dopamine D2 receptors; their antagonism at these receptors is related to their clinical antipsychotic potencies. It is the antidopaminergic action on the mesolimbic–mesocortical pathway that is believed to be the effect required for this clinical action.

A True

The antidopaminergic action on the nigrostriatal pathway causes extrapyramidal symptoms:

* parkinsonism
* dystonias
* akathisia
* tardive dyskinesia.

B False

Pyrexia may result from central antimuscarinic actions.

C True

The antidopaminergic action on the tuberoinfundibular pathway causes hormonal side-effects. Hyperprolactinaemia, resulting from the fact that dopamine is prolactin-inhibitory factor, causes:

* galactorrhoea
* gynaecomastia
* menstrual disturbances
* ↓ sperm count
* ↓ libido.

D False

This may result from antiadrenergic actions.

E False

While a reduction in libido may result from central antidopaminergic actions, ejaculatory failure in men may result in particular from antiadrenergic actions.

References/Further Reading

Revision Notes in Psychiatry, pp. 166–7.

17.3

In the central nervous system, MAO-A (monoamine oxidase type A) acts on:

- noradrenaline
- serotonin
- dopamine
- tyramine.

A True

B True

C True

D True

E False

In the central nervous system, MAO-B (monoamine oxidase type B) acts on:

- dopamine
- tyramine
- phenylethylamine
- benzylamine.

References/Further Reading

Revision Notes in Psychiatry, p. 168.

17.4

Lithium ions, Li$^+$, are monovalent cations that cause a number of effects, some of which may account for its therapeutic actions, including:

- ↑ intracellular Na$^+$
- ↓ Na,K-ATPase pump activity
- ↑ intracellular Ca^{2+} in erythrocytes in mania and depression
- ↑ erythrocyte choline
- ↑ erythrocyte phospholipid catabolism (via phospholipase D)
- ↓ Ca^{2+} in platelets in bipolar disorder
- ↑ serotonergic neurotransmission
- ↓ central 5-HT$_1$ and 5-HT$_2$ receptor density (demonstrated in the hippocampus)
- ↑ dopamine turnover in hypothalamic-tuberoinfundibular dopaminergic neurones
- ↓ central dopamine synthesis (dose-dependent)
- normalization of low plasma and CSF levels of GABA in bipolar disorder
- ↑ GABAergic neurotransmission
- ↓ low affinity GABA receptors in the corpus striatum and hypothalamus (chronic lithium administration)
- ↑ met-enkephalin and leu-enkephalin in the basal ganglia and nucleus accumbens
- ↑ dynorphin in the corpus striatum.

A False

Chronic lithium treatment leads to an increase in erythrocyte choline levels by more than 10-fold, probably because of lithium-induced:

- inhibition of choline transport
- increased phospholipase D-mediated breakdown of choline-containing phospholipids.

B False

Both acute and chronic lithium treatment have been found to cause an inhibition of Na,K-ATPase activity in central and peripheral neurones.

C True

D True

E True

References/Further Reading

Revision Notes in Psychiatry, p. 167.

17.5

Peripherally, most tricyclic antidepressants have an antimuscarinic action, which gives rise to peripheral antimuscarinic side-effects such as :

- dry mouth
- blurred vision
- urinary retention
- constipation.

A True

B False

Weight gain is a side-effect of tricyclic antidepressants, but is not the result of the antimuscarinic action. Some of the factors that may be involved in causing weight gain include:

- antihistaminic actions
- α-adrenoceptor-blocking actions
- tricyclic antidepressant-induced slowing of metabolism.

C True

D False

E True

References/Further Reading

Revision Notes in Psychiatry, p. 168.

17.6

A True

This is the most important postulated mode of action in the brain for the anxiolytic and sedative-hypnotic actions of benzodiazepines.

B False

The most important postulated mode of action in the brain of the azaspirodecanedione buspirone in achieving central therapeutic effects is partial agonism at 5-HT$_{1A}$ receptors.

C False

The most important postulated mode of action of propranolol in achieving anxiolytic effects is antagonism at peripheral β-adrenoceptors.

D True

The cyclopyrrolone zopiclone is believed to achieve a central hypnotic effect by acting on the same receptors as do benzodiazepines.

E True

The imidazopyridine zolpidem in believed to achieve a central hypnotic effect by acting on the same receptors as do benzodiazepines.

References/Further Reading

Revision Notes in Psychiatry, p. 169.

17.7

A True

Sodium valproate may achieve its anticonvulsant effect on the basis of the following actions:

- ↑ GABA
  - – ↓ GABA breakdown
  - – ↑ GABA release
  - – ↓ GABA turnover
  - – ↑ GABA-B receptor density
  - – ↑ neuronal responsiveness to GABA
- ↓ Na⁺ influx
- ↑ K⁺ conductance.

B False

The mode of action of gabapentin is not clear at the time of writing, but it is believed that it may act by binding to a cerebral calcium channel.

C True

Vigabatrin is believed to achieve its anticonvulsant effect by irreversibly inhibiting GABA transaminase.

D False

Lamotrigine is believed to achieve its anticonvulsant effect by inhibiting glutamate release and prolonging the slow inactivated state of voltage-dependent sodium ion channels.

E True

The antiepileptic actions of tiagabine are believed to result from the inhibition of neuronal and glial uptake of GABA.

References/Further Reading

Revision Notes in Psychiatry, pp. 169–70.

17.8

A True

ECT probably leads to increased noradrenergic function. In particular, ECT causes:

- ↑ cerebral noradrenaline activity
- ↑ cerebral tyrosine hydroxylase activity
- ↑ plasma catecholamines, particularly adrenaline.

B True

ECT probably leads to increased serotonergic function. In particular, ECT causes an acute:

- ↑ cerebral serotonin concentration.

C True

ECT probably leads to increased dopaminergic function. In particular, ECT causes an acute:

- ↑ cerebral dopamine concentration
- ↑ cerebral concentration of dopamine metabolites
- ↑ behavioural responsiveness to dopamine agonists.

D False

ECT probably leads to decreased central cholinergic function. In particular, ECT causes an acute:

- ↓ cerebral acetylcholine concentration
- ↑ cerebral acetyltransferase activity
- ↑ cerebral acetylcholinesterase activity
- ↑ CSF acetylcholine concentration.

E True

ECT has been shown to be associated with an acute increase in the release of GABA and with an acute increase in $GABA_B$ binding.

References/Further Reading

Revision Notes in Psychiatry, pp. 170–1.

Answers

18.1

Allergic reactions to drugs involve the body's immune system, with the drug interacting with a protein to form an immunogen that causes sensitization and the induction of an immune response. Criteria suggesting an allergic reaction include:

- a different time-course from that of the pharmacodynamic action, for example:
  - delayed onset of the adverse drug reaction
  - the adverse drug reaction manifests only after repeated drug exposure
- there may be no dose-related effect, with subtherapeutically small doses leading to sensitization or allergic reactions
- a hypersensitivity reaction, unrelated to the pharmacological actions of the drug, occurs.

A False

B True

C False

D False

The adverse drug reaction can occur with subtherapeutic doses of the drug in an allergic reaction.

E True

References/Further Reading

Revision Notes in Psychiatry, pp. 172–3.

18.2

Types of allergic reaction to drugs include:

- anaphylactic shock – type I hypersensitivity reaction
- haematological reactions – type II, III or IV hypersensitivity reaction; for example
  - haemolytic anaemia
  - agranulocytosis
  - thrombocytopenia
- allergic liver damage – type II ± III hypersensitivity reaction
- skin rashes – type IV hypersensitivity reaction
- generalized autoimmune (systemic lupus erythematosus-like) disease – type IV hypersensitivity reaction.

A False

This is a type I hypersensitivity reaction.

B True

C True

D False

E True

References/Further Reading

Revision Notes in Psychiatry, p. 173.

18.3

Neuroleptic malignant syndrome is characterized by:

- hyperthermia
- fluctuating level of consciousness
- muscular rigidity
- autonomic dysfunction
    - tachycardia
    - labile blood pressure
    - pallor
    - sweating
    - urinary incontinence.

Laboratory investigations commonly, but not invariably, demonstrate:

- ↑ creatinine phosphokinase
- ↑ white blood count
- abnormal liver function tests.

Neuroleptic malignant syndrome requires urgent medical treatment.

A True

B True

C False

D False

E True

References/Further Reading

Revision Notes in Psychiatry, p. 174.

18.4

Long-term high-dose pharmacotherapy with chlorpromazine may cause ocular and skin changes, such as:

- opacity of the lens
- opacity of the cornea
- purplish pigmentation of the skin
- purplish pigmentation of the conjunctiva
- purplish pigmentation of the cornea
- purplish pigmentation of the retina.

A True

B False

C True

D True

E True

References/Further Reading

Revision Notes in Psychiatry, p. 174.

18.5

A False

This is not a sensitivity reaction.

B True

C True

D True

E True

References/Further Reading

Revision Notes in Psychiatry, p. 174.

18.6

Clozapine may cause neutropenia and potentially fatal agranulocytosis, because of which regular haematological monitoring is required. Other side-effects of clozapine include hypersalivation and side-effects common to chlorpromazine, including extrapyramidal symptoms.

A True

B True

This is potentially fatal.

C True

This should be evaluated in order to rule out an underlying infection or agranulocytosis. Patients should be instructed to report any symptoms of infection immediately.

D True

Pharmacotherapy with clozapine should be discontinued immediately if the patient develops jaundice.

E True

References/Further Reading

Revision Notes in Psychiatry, p. 174.

18.7

A True

These drugs may cause antimuscarinic side-effects.

B False

There may be a worsening of tardive dyskinesia.

C True

D True

E False

Antimuscarinic drugs are useful in reducing sialorrhoea.

References/Further Reading

Revision Notes in Psychiatry, p. 175.

18.8

A False

The therapeutic index of a drug is inversely proportional to the therapeutic dose of the drug.

B True

C True

The therapeutic index of lithium is low (narrow) and therefore regular plasma lithium level monitoring is required.

D False

E True

Newer antidepressants generally have a higher (wider) therapeutic index and are therefore safer in overdose.

References/Further Reading

Revision Notes in Psychiatry, p. 175.

18.9

The lithium dose should be adjusted to achieve a lithium level of 0.4–1.0 mmol L^{-1} for prophylactic purposes, with lower levels being used in the elderly. Side-effects of lithium therapy in its therapeutic range include:

- fatigue
- drowsiness
- dry mouth
- a metallic taste
- polydipsia
- polyuria
- nausea
- vomiting
- weight gain
- diarrhoea
- fine tremor
- muscle weakness
- oedema.

A True

Oedema should not be treated with diuretics because thiazide and loop diuretics reduce lithium excretion and can thereby cause lithium intoxication.

B False

Polyuria is a side-effect of lithium in its therapeutic range. Oliguria is seen in severe lithium overdosage.

C True

D False

A fine tremor is a side-effect of lithium in its therapeutic range. A coarse tremor is a sign of lithium intoxication.

E True

References/Further Reading

Revision Notes in Psychiatry, p. 175.

18.10

Signs of lithium intoxication include:

- mild drowsiness and sluggishness $\rightarrow$ giddiness and ataxia
- lack of coordination
- blurred vision
- tinnitus
- anorexia
- dysarthria
- vomiting
- diarrhoea
- coarse tremor
- muscle weakness.

A True

B True

C True

D False

This is a sign of severe overdosage of lithium. At lithium plasma levels of greater than 2 mmol L^{-1} the following effects can occur:

- hyperreflexia and hyperextension of the limbs
- toxic psychoses
- convulsions
- syncope
- oliguria
- circulatory failure
- coma
- death.

E True

References/Further Reading

Revision Notes in Psychiatry, p. 175.

18.11

All true.

Long-term treatment with lithium may give rise to:

- thyroid function disturbances
  - goitre
  - hypothyroidism
- memory impairment
- nephrotoxicity
- cardiovascular changes
  - T-wave flattening on the ECG
  - arrhythmias.

   Thyroid function tests are usually carried out routinely every 6 months in order to check for lithium-induced disturbances.

References/Further Reading

Revision Notes in Psychiatry, p. 176.

18.12

A True

Allergic and haematological reactions to tricyclic antidepressants include:

- agranulocytosis
- leucopenia
- eosinophilia
- thrombocytopenia
- skin rash
- photosensitization
- facial oedema
- allergic cholestatic jaundice.

B False

Testicular enlargement is a side-effect.

C True

D True

This results from blockade of α_1-adrenoceptors.

E True

References/Further Reading

Revision Notes in Psychiatry, pp. 176–7.

18.13

The inhibition of peripheral pressor amines, particularly dietary tryramine, by MAOIs can lead to a hypertensive crisis when foodstuffs rich in tyramine are eaten. Foods that should therefore be avoided when on treatment with MAOIs include:

- cheese – except cottage cheese and cream cheese
- meat extracts and yeast extracts
- alcohol – particularly chianti, fortified wines and beer
- non-fresh fish
- non-fresh meat
- non-fresh poultry
- offal
- avocado
- banana skins
- broad-bean pods
- caviar
- herring – pickled or smoked.

A True

B False

In general, cheese contains a significant amount of amines (particularly tyramine) per unit mass, so that it should be avoided by patients taking MAOIs. This does not apply, however, to cottage cheese or cream cheese.

C True

D True

E False

It is safe to drink milk but cheese (cooked or plain) should be avoided (apart from the types mentioned in B above).

References/Further Reading

Puri, B.K. and Sklar, J. (1990) *Revision for the MRCPsych Part I*. Edinburgh: Churchill Livingstone, pp. 105–6.
Revision Notes in Psychiatry, pp. 177–8.

18.14

Medicines that should be avoided by patients taking MAOIs include:

- indirectly acting sympathomimetic amines, e.g.
  - amphetamine
  - fenfluramine
  - ephedrine
  - phenylpropanolamine
- cough mixtures containing sympathomimetics
- nasal decongestants containing sympathomimetics
- L-dopa
- pethidine
- tricyclic antidepressants.

A False

B True

C True

D False

E True

The combination of tranylcypromine with clomipramine is particularly dangerous.

References/Further Reading

Revision Notes in Psychiatry, p. 178.

18.15

The more important side-effects of benzodiazepines include:

• anxiety (probably a rebound effect)
• confusion and ataxia (particularly in the elderly)
• drowsiness
• physical dependence
• psychological impairment.

   Other side-effects that occur occasionally include:

• changes in libido
• changes in salivation
• hypotension
• rashes
• urinary retention.

A True

B True

C False

Respiratory depression is a side-effect.

D True

E True

If benzodiazepines are taken regularly for 4 weeks or more, dependence may develop, so that sudden cessation of intake may then lead to a withdrawal syndrome whose main features include:
• anxiety symptoms
    – palpitations
    – tremor
    – panic
    – dizziness
    – nausea
    – sweating
    – other somatic symptoms
• low mood
• abnormal experiences
    – depersonalization
    – derealization
    – hypersensitivity to sensations in all modalities
    – distorted perception of space
    – tinnitus
    – formication
    – a strange taste
• influenza-like symptoms

- psychiatric/neurological symptoms
  - epileptic seizures
  - confusional states
  - psychotic episodes
- insomnia
- loss of appetite
- weight loss.

References/Further Reading

Puri, B.K. and Sklar, J. (1990) *Revision for the MRCPsych Part I*. Edinburgh: Churchill
   Livingstone, pp. 99–100.
Revision Notes in Psychiatry, pp. 178–9.

18.16

If alcohol is drunk while disulfiram is being taken regularly, acetaldehyde accumulates. Thus, ingesting even small amounts of alcohol then causes unpleasant systemic reactions, including:

- facial flushing
- headache
- palpitations
- tachycardia
- nausea
- vomiting.

Ingestion of large amounts of alcohol while being treated with disulfiram can lead to:

- air hunger
- arrhythmias
- severe hypotension.

A False

Disulfiram causes the inhibition of aldehyde dehydrogenase, an enzyme involved in the metabolism of ethanol. Following the ingestion of ethanol, acetaldehyde accumulates.

B True

C False

D True

E True

References/Further Reading

Revision Notes in Psychiatry, p. 179.

18.17

Side-effects of this antiandrogen agent in men include:

* inhibition of spermatogenesis
* tiredness
* gynaecomastia
* weight gain
* improvement of existing acne vulgaris
* ↑ scalp hair growth
* female pattern of pubic hair growth.

Liver function tests should be carried out regularly because of a theoretical risk to the liver. Dyspnoea may result from high-dose treatment.

A True

B False
Existing acne vulgaris often improves.

C False

D False
Tiredness is a side-effect.

E True

References/Further Reading

Revision Notes in Psychiatry, p. 179.

Answers

19.1

Meiosis occurs in gametogenesis via the following stages

- interphase
- prophase I
- metaphase I
- anaphase I
- telophase I
- prophase II
- metaphase II
- anaphase II
- telophase II.

A False

Meiosis involves two stages of cell division.

B False

Chromosomal division takes place once during meiosis.

C True

As chromosomal division takes place once, the resulting gametes are haploid.

D False

Recombination takes place duing prophase I.

E True

References/Further Reading

Revision Notes in Psychiatry, p. 183.

19.2

Genes, the biological units of heredity, consist of codons grouped into exons with intervening nucleotide sequences known as introns. The introns do not code for amino acids. Genes also contain nucleotide sequences at their beginning and end that allow transcription to take place accurately. Thus, starting from the 5' end (upstream), a typical eukaryotic gene contains the following:

- upstream site-regulating transcription
- promoter (TATA)
- transcription initiation site
- 5' non-coding region
- exons
- introns
- 3' non-coding region, containing a poly A addition site.

A False

B True

C False

It is 'downstream'.

D True

E True

References/Further Reading

Revision Notes in Psychiatry, p. 183.

19.3

A karyotype is an arrangement of the chromosomal make-up of somatic cells that can be produced by carrying out the following procedures in turn:

- arrest cell division at an appropriate stage
- disperse the chromosomes
- fix the chromosomes
- stain the chromosomes
- photograph the chromosomes
- identify the chromosomes
- arrange the chromosomes.

A True

B True

C False

D False

E False

This is a technique that allows the transfer of DNA fragments from gel, where electrophoresis and DNA denaturation have taken place, to a nylon or nitrocellular filter. It involves overlaying the gel with the filter and in turn overlaying the filter with paper towels. A solution is then blotted through the gel to the paper towels. Autoradiography can then be used to identify the fragments of interest on the filter. The technique is named after its inventor, Edwin Southern.

References/Further Reading

Revision Notes in Psychiatry, pp. 182 and 187.

19.4

Transcription is the step in gene expression in which information from the DNA molecule is transcibed onto a primary RNA transcript. This is followed by splicing and nuclear transport, so that the information (minus that from introns) then exists in the cytoplasm of the cell on mRNA (messenger RNA).

Following transcription, splicing and nuclear transport, translation is the process in gene expression whereby mRNA acts as a template allowing the genetic code to be deciphered to allow the formation of a peptide chain. This process involves tRNA molecules.

A False

tRNAs are involved in translation but not transcription.

B False

Ultimately, in humans, there is just left an mRNA template based on the exons; the 'information' from introns is spliced out.

C False

Uniparental disomy refers to the phenomenon in which an individual inherits both homologues of a chromosome pair from the same parent.

D True

E False

References/Further Reading

Revision Notes in Psychiatry, pp. 183 and 185.

19.5

A False

This is the law of segregation. It is Mendel's second law that is the law of independent assortment.

B False

Autosomal dominant disorders result from the presence of an abnormal dominant allele causing the individual to manifest the abnormal phenotypic trait. Features of autosomal dominant transmission include:

- the phenotypic trait is present in all individuals carrying the dominant allele
- the phenotypic trait does not skip generations – vertical transmission takes place
- men and women are affected
- male to male transmission can take place
- transmission is not solely dependent on parental consanguineous matings
- if one parent is homozgyous for the abnormal dominant allele, all the members of F1 will manifest the abnormal phenotypic trait.

Variable expressivity can cause clinical features of autosomal dominant disorders to vary between affected individuals. This, together with reduced penetrance, may give the appearance that the disorder has skipped a generation. The sudden appearance of an autosomal dominant disorder may occur as a result of a new dominant mutation.

C True

Autosomal recessive disorders result from the presence of two abnormal recessive alleles causing the individual to manifest the abnormal phenotypic trait. Features of autosomal recessive transmission include:

- heterozygous individuals are generally carriers who do not manifest the abnormal phenotypic trait
- the rarer the disorder the more likely it is that the parents are consanguineous
- the disorder tends to miss generations but the affected individuals in a family tend to be found among siblings – horizontal transmission takes place.

D False

In X-linked recessive disorders a recessive abnormal allele is carried on the X chromosome. All male (XY) offspring inheriting this allele manifest the abnormal phenotypic trait. Other features of X-linked recessive transmission include:

- Male to male transmission does not take place.
- Female heterozygotes are carriers.

E True

In X-linked dominant disorders a dominant abnormal allele is carried on the X chromosome. If an affected male mates with an unaffected female, all the daughters and none of the sons are affected. If an unaffected male mates with an affected heterozygous female, half the daughters and half the sons, on average, are affected. Male-to-male transmission does not take place.

References/Further Reading

Revision Notes in Psychiatry, pp. 184–5.

19.6

A DNA polymorphism, such as a restriction fragment length polymorphism, if linked to a given disease locus, can be used as a genetic marker in linkage analysis without its precise chromosomal location being known. Genetic markers can also be used in presymptomatic diagnosis and prenatal diagnosis. (Restriction fragment length polymorphisms, or RFLPs, are polymorphisms at restriction enzyme cleavage sites that give rise to fragments of different lengths following restriction enzyme digestion. They can be used as DNA markers and are usually inherited in a simple Mendelian fashion.)

A True

B False

This refers to the phenomenon in which an allele is differentially expressed depending on whether it is maternally or paternally derived.

C True

D True

E False

Restriction enzymes, also known as restriction endonucleases, cleave DNA only at locations containing specific nucleotide sequences. Different restriction enzymes target different nucleotide sequences, but a given restriction enzyme targets the same sequence. (These enzymes are not synthesized using genetic markers.)

References/Further Reading

Revision Notes in Psychiatry, pp. 185, 187–8.

19.7

Linkage is the phenomenon whereby two genes close to each other on the same chromosome are likely to be inherited together. The recombinant fraction is a measure of how often the alleles at two loci are separated during meiotic recombination. The value of the recombinant fraction can vary from zero to 0.5. The lod score for a given recombinant fraction is the logarithm to base 10 of the odds $P_1:P_2$, where P_1 is the probability of there being linkage for a given recombinant fraction and P_2 is the probability of there being no measurable linkage. Thus the lod score gives a measure of the probability of two loci being linked. The lod score method was devised by Morton.

A False

The logarithm to base 10 rather than the natural logarithm (i.e. the logarithm to base e) is used in the calculation of the lod score.

B True

C True

D False

In molecular genetics, the maximum likelihood score is the value of the recombinant fraction that gives the highest value for the lod score. It represents the best estimate that can be made for the recombinant fraction from the given available data.

E True

References/Further Reading

Revision Notes in Psychiatry, p. 188.

19.8

A True

Approximately 95% of cases of Down's syndrome result from trisomy 21 following non-disjunction during meiosis.

B True

Approximately 4% of cases of Down's syndrome result from translocation involving chromosome 21.

C True

D False

It is trisomy 21 that accounts for most cases of this disorder.

E True

Cases of the disorder that are not caused by either trisomy 21 following non-disjunction during meiosis or translocation involving chromosome 21 are mosaics.

References/Further Reading

Revision Notes in Psychiatry, p. 188.

19.9

A False

This is caused by trisomy 18, i.e. 47, +18.

B True

This is caused by trisomy 13.

C False

This results from the partial deletion of the short arm of chromosome 5. The characteristic kitten-like cry has been localized to 5p15.3, while other clinical features have been localized to 5p15.2 (the cri-du-chat critical region of CDCCR).

D False

In this syndrome the genotype of phenotypic women is 47,XXX. The genotype 48,XXXY occurs in Klinefelter's syndrome; the most common genotype in Klinefelter's syndrome is 47,XXY.

E True

This genotype is also written as 45,XO.

References/Further Reading

Revision Notes in Psychiatry, pp. 188–9.

19.10

A False

This is an autosomal recessive disorder of carbohydrate metabolism.

B False

This is also an autosomal recessive disorder of carbohydrate metabolism.

C True

D True

This is one of the phacomatoses.

E True

This is also one of the phacomatoses.

References/Further Reading

Revision Notes in Psychiatry, p. 189.

19.11

A True

In this amino aciduria there is renal loss and impaired intestinal absorption of the following amino acids:

- cystine
- ornithine
- arginine
- lysine.

B True

Citrullinaemia (arginosuccinic acid synthetase deficiency) is a urea cycle disorder.

C True

In this autosomal recessive disorder a deficiency of branched-chain ketoacid dehydrogenase leads to an impaired ability to metabolize the branched-chain oxoacids of the following amino acids:

- leucine
- isoleucine
- valine.

D False

This is one of the phacomatoses and it can be inherited in an autosomal dominant manner.

E False

This is a disorder of carbohydrate metabolism rather than of protein metabolism.

References/Further Reading

Revision Notes in Psychiatry, pp. 189–90.

19.12

A True

This is a sphingolipidosis or lysosomal storage disease.

B False

Hunter syndrome (mucopolysaccharidosis type II) is inherited as an X-linked recessive disorder.

C True

D False

Wilson disease is not a disorder of carbohydrate metabolism.

E True

There is a deficiency of the enzyme fructose 1-phosphate aldolase.

References/Further Reading

Revision Notes in Psychiatry, p. 190.

19.13

A True

In this X-linked disorder (chromosomal location Xq26–q27.2) there is a deficiency of the enzyme hypoxanthine guanine phosphoribosyltransferase leading to an inability to retrieve the following purines:

- hypoxanthine
- guanine.

  This is turn leads to an increased production of uric acid and therefore to hyperuricaemia.

B True

A fragile site occurs at Xq27.3.

C True

The chromosomal location of this disorder is Xq26.1.

D False

This is an X-linked dominant disorder.

E True

References/Further Reading

Revision Notes in Psychiatry, p. 191.

Answers

20.1

The prevalence of a disease (or disorder) is the proportion of a defined population that has the disease at a given point in time. The population used may be defined variously, for example in terms of demography, geography, in relation to index cases of the same of another disease, and in relation to social, psychological, genetic and environmental factors. For example, one may wish to study the prevalence of a given psychiatric disorder in the sons of alcoholic mothers.

A True

The point prevalence is the proportion of a defined population that has a given disease at a given point in time, and is obtained by dividing the number of people having the disease at the given point in time by the total population at that same point in time.

B False

The population at risk of a given disease is the population of individuals free of a given disease, who have not already had the disease by the time of the commencement of the specified time period; instead, it includes only individuals free of the disease who are at risk of becoming new cases.

C True

The lifetime prevalence is the proportion of a defined population that has or has had a given disease (at any time during each person's lifetime so far) at a given point in time.

D True

The disease rate at post mortem is the proportion of bodies on which post mortems are carried out that has a given disease. It is a measure of prevalence.

E True

The birth defect rate is the proportion of live births that has a given disease. The birth defect rate is a type of prevalence and not a measure of incidence.

References/Further Reading

Revision Notes in Psychiatry, p. 192.
Sciences Basic to Psychiatry, 2nd edn, pp. 303–4.

20.2

The incidence of a disease is the rate of occurrence of new cases in a defined population over a given period of time.

A False

The units given in the question do not include a temporal component; while 'per 100 000' is incorrect, 'per 100 000 per year' is a unit of incidence. In general, the unit of incidence is (specified time period)$^{-1}$. For example, the incidence of schizophrenia published by Dunham in 1965 was approximately 0.22 per 1000 per year (or 22 per 100 000 per year).

B True

The morbidity rate of a disease is the rate of occurrence of new non-fatal cases of the disease in a defined population at risk over a given period of time. It is a measurement of incidence and therefore has the same units as incidence.

C True

The mortality rate is the number of deaths in a defined population during a given period of time divided by the number in the population during the same time period. For the mortality rate from a given disease, the numerator of the ratio is replaced by the number of deaths from that disease. As with the morbidity rate, the mortality rate is a measurement of incidence and therefore has the same units as incidence.

D False

In the steady state, in which the incidence of a disease remains constant during a given period of time, and the time between the onset of caseness (the time of diagnosis) and its ending (at recovery or death) also remains constant, the point prevalence, P, of the disease is directly proportional to the incidence, I

$$P = ID$$

where D is the chronicity or average duration of the disease.

E False

The incidence of a disease is calculated by dividing the number of new cases over the given time period by the total population at risk during the same time period. As mentioned in the answer to the previous question, the population at risk does not include people who have already had the disease by the time of the commencement of the specified time period; instead, it includes only individuals free of the disease who are at risk of becoming new cases. In calculating the incidence, individuals who have already had the disease (and therefore cannot become new cases) must also be excluded from the numerator.

References/Further Reading

Revision Notes in Psychiatry, p. 192.
Sciences Basic to Psychiatry, 2nd edn, p. 304.

20.3

A True

Because it is a ratio of two numbers, prevalence does not have any units, and may be expressed as a percentage by multiplication by 100. For example, Jablensky and Sartorius in 1975 estimated the annual prevalence (a period prevalence) of schizophrenia to be 2–4 per 1000 (or 0.2–0.4%).

B False

The chronicity or average duration of a disease is measured in units of time (e.g. months, years). It therefore has the inverse units of the incidence of the disease. For example, if the incidence is the rate per year, then the chronicity is measured in years.

C True

The relative risk is the ratio of two incidences and therefore does not have any units.

D True

E True

The standardized mortality ratio, conventionally abbreviated to SMR, is the ratio of the observed standardized mortality rate (from the population under study) to the expected standardized mortality rate (from the standard population), and is usually expressed as a percentage by multiplying this ratio by 100.

References/Further Reading

Sciences Basic to Psychiatry, 2nd edn, pp. 304–5.
Revision Notes in Psychiatry, pp. 192–3.

20.4

The standardized mortality rate is the mortality rate adjusted to compensate for a confounder.

A True

B False
This is part of the calculation; it is not taken into account 'sometimes'.

C True

D True

E False
This has already taken age into account.

References/Further Reading

Sciences Basic to Psychiatry, 2nd edn, pp. 304–305.
Revision Notes in Psychiatry, pp. 192–193.

20.5

The relative risk of a disease with respect to a given risk factor is the ratio of the incidence of the disease in people exposed to that risk factor to the incidence of the disease in people not exposed to the same risk factor.

A False

A value of 1 for the relative risk implies no causation, and this is the null hypothesis in hypothesis testing.

B False

The association is positive if the relative risk is greater than 1, and negative if it is less than 1.

C True

D True

When the relative risk has a value that is statistically significantly different to 1, this is taken as evidence of an association between the disease and the relevant risk factor.

E True

References/Further Reading

Sciences Basic to Psychiatry, 2nd edn, pp. 304–5.
Revision Notes in Psychiatry, pp. 192–3.

20.6

A True

B False

The relative risk of a disease with respect to a given risk factor is the ratio of the incidence of the disease in people exposed to that risk factor to the incidence of the disease in people not exposed to the same risk factor. The incidence of the disease in people exposed to the risk factor is $a/(a + b)$, and the incidence of the disease in people not exposed to the risk factor is $c/(c + d)$. Therefore the relative risk is the former divided by the latter:

relative risk $= a(c + d)/[c(a + b)]$

C True

D False

Odds ratio $= ad/(bc)$.

E True

The attributable risk, also known as the risk difference or absolute excess risk, is the incidence of the disease in the group exposed to the risk factor being studied minus the incidence of the disease in the group not exposed to this risk factor. Hence:

attributable risk $= a/(a + b) - c/(c + d)$

References/Further Reading

Sciences Basic to Psychiatry, 2nd edn, pp. 304–5.
Revision Notes in Psychiatry, pp. 192–3.

20.7

The morbidity rate of a disease is the rate of occurrence of new non-fatal cases of the disease in a defined population at risk over a given period of time.

A True

B True

C False

Non-fatal cases need to be measured in determining morbidity rates.

D True

E True

References/Further Reading

Sciences Basic to Psychiatry, 2nd edn, p. 305.
Revision Notes in Psychiatry, p. 193.

20.8

The development of psychiatric assessment instruments, such as standardized psychiatric interview schedules and screening questionnaires, have greatly aided the identification of cases for research purposes. A commonly used standardized psychiatric interview schedule developed in Britain is the Present State Examination (PSE) (Wing *et al.*, 1974).

A False

The PSE consists of a 140-item semi-structured interview, with probes being suggested for individual symptoms.

B True

The results of the PSE can be entered into a computer program called CATEGO, which then provides a CATEGO and ICD-9 classification.

C True

The PSE is particularly useful in the diagnosis of schizophrenia.

D False

The PSE has a poor reliability so far as the diagnosis of personality disorder, organicity, alcoholism and mental retardation are concerned.

E True

While the PSE is primarily a diagnostic instrument, a development of it known as the Index of Definition (ID) can be used to identify cases of psychiatric disorder. The PSE data are used to assign an ID between one (no symptoms) and eight, with an ID of five being the threshold for caseness. If an individual scores five or more, then the PSE data can be used to give a diagnosis.

References/Further Reading

Sciences Basic to Psychiatry, 2nd edn, p. 307.
Revision Notes in Psychiatry, p. 192.
Wing, J.K., Cooper, J.E. and Sartorius, N. (1974) *The Measurement and Classification of Psychiatric Symptoms.* London: Cambridge University Press.

20.9

The General Health Questionnaire (GHQ) is a questionnaire commonly used for screening for psychiatric disorder.

A True

The GHQ consists of 60 items each with four possible answers.

B False

It is self-rated.

C False

It was devised by Goldberg (1972). Wing was responsible for the development of the PSE (see previous question).

D False

The GHQ is not meant to be used to identify psychotic cases.

E True

References/Further Reading

Sciences Basic to Psychiatry, 2nd edn, p. 307.
Revision Notes in Psychiatry, p. 192.
Goldberg, D.P. (1972) *The Detection of Psychiatric Illness by Questionnaire. Maudsley Monograph 21*. London: Oxford University Press.

20.10

The sensitivity and specificity of an assessment instrument or any other test give a measure of its effectiveness. They are functions of the test and not of the tested individuals. Sensitivity and specificity are measures of the true positive and true negative rates respectively.

A False

>   Sensitivity = true positive/(true positive + false negative)

Therefore the sensitivity of the test is $a/(a + c)$.

The sensitivity of a test is often expressed as a percentage by multiplying the above expression by 100. It can be seen from this expression that the sensitivity of a test is an index of how well it detects what is being looked for.

B False

>   Specificity = true negative/(true negative + false positive)

Therefore the specificity of the test is $d/(d + b)$

The specificity of a test is expressed as a percentage by multiplying the above expression by 100. It can be seen from this expression that the specificity of a test is an index of how well what is not being looked for (true negatives) is excluded.

C True

The predictive value of a positive test result is the proportion of the positive results that is true positive, i.e. $a/(a + b)$. It is often expressed as a percentage by multiplying this expression by 100.

D True

The predictive value of a negative test result is the proportion of the negative results that is true negative, i.e. $d/(d + c) = d/(c + d)$. It is often expressed as a percentage by multiplying this expression by 100.

E False

The efficiency of a test is the proportion of all the results that is true (true positive or true negative), i.e. $(a + d)/(a + b + c + d)$. It is often expressed as a percentage by multiplying this expression by 100.

References/Further Reading

Sciences Basic to Psychiatry, 2nd edn, p. 307–8.
Revision Notes in Psychiatry, p. 192.

Answers

Note that many of the questions in this chapter refer in particular to British law.

21.1

If a person lacking capacity has little capital and receives income only from state benefits, the necessary financial arrangements can be made under regulation 33 of the Social Security (Claims and Payments) Regulations 1987, which provides that the Secretary of State may appoint someone, the appointee, to act on behalf of the claimant.

A False

The appointee has no power to deal with the claimant's capital.

B True

C False

The appointee must be aged 18 or over.

D True

E True

References/Further Reading

Jones, R.M. (1996) *Mental Health Act Manual*, 5th edn. London: Sweet & Maxwell, pp. 286–7.
Revision Notes in Psychiatry, p. 194.

21.2

A power of attorney is a means whereby one person (the donor) gives legal authority to another person (the attorney) to manage his or her affairs.

A False

The attorney is not an advocate; he or she has no legal status.

B True

C False

When the donor loses their mental capacity to manage their own affairs, then an ordinary power of attorney is automatically revoked.

D False

Regulation is carried out by the Public Trust Office.

E True

References/Further Reading

Jones, R.M. (1996) *Mental Health Act Manual*, 5th edn. London: Sweet & Maxwell, pp. 287–8.
Revision Notes in Psychiatry, p. 194.

21.3

A False

Testamentary capacity is the ability to make a valid will.

B True

As a reaction against the fact that mentally disordered people were still being hanged despite the McNaughten Rules (which came into being after McNaughten, while deluded, attempted to shoot Sir Robert Peel in 1843), a movement was created to bring in a defence of diminished responsibility, i.e. the responsibility of the offender is not totally absent because of mental abnormality, but is only partially impaired. As a result, the offender would be found guilty but the sentence would be modified. This was made law in the Homicide Act 1957, and applies only to charges of murder. Under Section 2 of the Homicide Act 1957, the offender may plead that, at the time of the offence, he or she had diminished responsibility. The offender has to show that, at the material time, he or she suffered from 'such abnormality of mind, whether caused by a condition of arrested or retarded development of mind, or any inherent causes, or induced by disease or injury, such that it substantially impaired his [or her] mental responsibility for his [or her] acts'.

C True

D False

The Court's powers are limited to dealing with the financial and legal affairs of the person concerned.

E False

A valid will is not invalidated by the subsequent impairment of testamentary capacity.

References/Further Reading

Revision Notes in Psychiatry, pp. 194–5.
Textbook of Psychiatry, pp. 371, 388–9.

21.4

A False

Medical evidence that any form of mental disorder has rendered a person incapable of managing his or her property and affairs can be put to a judge in the Court of Protection.

B True

C False

The receiver is often a relative, friend or solicitor. The receiver must keep accounts and spend the patient's money on things that will benefit the patient. The Court must give permission before the disposal of capital assets, such as the sale of property.

D False

Only one medical certificate is required, from a registered medical practitioner who has examined the patient. This registered medical practitioner does not necessarily have to be a doctor approved under the Mental Health Act.

E True

The patient should be given notice that an application has been made to the Court of Protection. He or she has until the hearing date, or 7 clear days (whichever is later), to write to the Court. The patient has the right to object, preferably with medical evidence, if he or she maintains that he or she is not incapable of managing his or her affairs.

References/Further Reading

Bluglass, R. (1983) *A Guide to the Mental Health Act 1983.* Edinburgh: Churchill Livingstone, p. 112.
Revision Notes in Psychiatry, pp. 194–5.
Textbook of Psychiatry, p. 400.

21.5

A False

The responsibility for making the decision about whether or not a person (including a psychiatric patient) should continue to drive is that of the Driver and Vehicle Licensing Authority (DVLA), with the doctor acting only as a source of information and advice.

B False

The driver has a duty to keep the DVLA informed of any condition that may impair his or her ability to drive.

C True

The patient's doctor is responsible for advising the patient to inform the DVLA of a condition likely to make driving dangerous. If the patient fails to take this advice, the doctor may then contact the DVLA directly.

D False

A driver with a Mobility Allowance may drive from the age of 16 years.

E True

References/Further Reading

Revision Notes in Psychiatry, p. 195.

21.6

Group 1 entitlement allows a person to drive a motor car or motor bike.

A False

The DVLA need not be notified and driving need not cease after suffering from an anxiety state. Patients must be warned about the possible effects of medication that may affect fitness. However, serious psychoneurotic episodes affecting or likely to affect driving should be notified to the DVLA and the patient should be advised not to drive.

B False

The DVLA need not be notified, and driving need not necessarily cease. Patients must be warned about the possible effects of medication that may affect fitness. However, serious psychoneurotic episodes affecting or likely to affect driving should be notified to the DVLA and the patient advised not to drive.

C True

The DVLA advises that, after an acute episode requiring hospital admission, the patient should be off the road for 6 months. Their licence is restored after freedom from symptoms during this period, and if the patient demonstrates that he the patient complies safely with the recommended medication and shows insight into his or her condition.

D True

The DVLA advises that, after an acute episode of hypomania requiring hospital admission, the patient should be off the road for 6–12 months, depending on the severity and frequency of relapses. The licence is restored after freedom from symptoms during this period, and if the patient demonstrates safe compliance with his or her medication.

E True

Severe mental handicap means a state of arrested or incomplete development of mind that includes a severe impairment of intelligence and social functioning. Severe mental handicap is a prescribed disability, and a licence must be refused or revoked.

References/Further Reading

Revision Notes in Psychiatry, pp. 196–7.

21.7

Group 2 entitlement is required for LGV/PCV driving.

A True

B True

C True

Any psychotropic medication necessary must be of low dosage and must not interfere with alertness or concentration or in any way impair driving performance.

D False

Pharmacotherapy during the 3 years following the hospital admission is not a criterion for rejecting an application for Group 2 entitlement.

E True

Consultant psychiatric examination is required before restoration of licence to confirm that there is no residual impairment and that the applicant has insight and would be able to recognize if he or she became unwell. There should be no significant likelihood of recurrence.

References/Further Reading

Revision Notes in Psychiatry, pp. 196–7.

21.8

Group 1 entitlement allows a person to drive a motor car or motor bike. In the following cases, independent medical assessment and urine screening, arranged by the DVLA, may be required.

A True

The regular use, confirmed by medical enquiry, will lead to licence revocation or refusal for a 6-month period.

B True

The regular use, confirmed by medical enquiry, will lead to licence revocation or refusal for a 6-month period.

C True

The regular use, confirmed by medical enquiry, will lead to licence revocation or refusal for a 6-month period.

D True

The regular use, or dependency on, benzodiazepines, confirmed by medical enquiry, will lead to licence revocation or refusal for a minimum 1-year period.

E True

The regular use, or dependency on, cocaine, confirmed by medical enquiry, will lead to licence revocation or refusal for a minimum 1-year period. In addition to benzodiazepines and cocaine, a similar situation applies to:

- amphetamines
- heroin
- morphine.

It also applies to morphine, except that applicants or drivers on consultant-supervised oral methadone-withdrawal programmes may be licensed, subject to annual medical review and favourable assessment.

References/Further Reading

Revision Notes in Psychiatry, pp. 201.

Note that the questions in this chapter refer to the Mental Health Act 1983 of England and Wales.

22.1

A False

The nearest relative is the first surviving person in the following list, with full blood relatives taking preference over half blood relatives, and the elder of two relatives of the same description or level of kinship also taking preference:

- husband or wife
- son or daughter
- father or mother
- brother or sister
- grandparent
- grandchild
- uncle or aunt
- nephew or niece.

Preference is also given to a relative with whom the patient ordinarily lives or by whom they are cared for.

B True

C False

The term mental illness is not formally defined in the Mental Health Act. Its operational definition is a matter of clinical judgement in each case.

D False

The term medical treatment includes nursing, and also includes care, habilitation and rehabilitation under medical supervision.

E True

References/Further Reading

Revision Notes in Psychiatry, pp. 202 and 204.

22.2

Under the Mental Health Act 1983, there is nothing in Subsection 2 of Section 1 of the Act that may be construed as implying that a person may be dealt with under this Act as suffering from mental disorder, or from any form of mental disorder described in this section, by reason only of:

- promiscuity
- other immoral conduct
- sexual deviancy
- dependence on alcohol
- dependence on drugs.

A False

B False

C True

D False

E False

References/Further Reading

Revision Notes in Psychiatry, p. 204.

22.3

Under Section 7, Subsection 2 of the Mental Health Act 1983, a guardianship application may be made in respect of a patient on the grounds that:

(a) he is suffering from mental disorder, i.e. mental illness, severe mental impairment, psychopathic disorder or mental impairment, and his mental disorder is of a nature or degree that warrants his reception into guardianship under this section; and

(b) it is necessary in the interests of the welfare of the patient or for the protection of other persons that the patient should be so received.

A False

A guardianship application shall be founded on the written recommendations in the prescribed form of two registered medical practitioners, including in each case a statement that, in the opinion of the practitioner, the conditions set out in Subsection (2) above are complied with.

B False

A patient may not be received into guardianship if they have not attained the age of 16 years.

C False

The person named as guardian in a guardianship application may be either a local social services authority or any other person (including the applicant).

D False

After approval, the application confers on the authority or person named in the application as guardian, to the exclusion of any other person, the power to require the patient to reside at a place specified by the authority or person named as guardian.

E False

The application may be made either by an approved social worker or by the nearest relative of the patient.

References/Further Reading

Mental Health Act 1983. Chapter 20. London: HMSO.

22.4

A True

B True

C False

The description is of Section 38 and is not a civil treatment order.

D False

This is Section 136.

E False

This is Section 135.

References/Further Reading

Revision Notes in Psychiatry, p. 203.

22.5

Section 57 covers irreversible, hazardous or non-established treatments.

A True

Section 57 covers any surgical operation for destroying brain tissue or for destroying the functioning of brain tissue.

B True

Section 57 covers hormone implants, e.g. for sex offenders.

C True

Section 57 covers potentially irreversible operations, such as castration.

D False

Electroconvulsive therapy is covered by Section 58 of the Mental Health Act 1983.

E False

References/Further Reading

Revision Notes in Psychiatry, p. 204.

22.6

A True

B True

C False
This is Section 35 of the Mental Health Act.

D True

E True

References/Further Reading

Revision Notes in Psychiatry, pp. 205–6.

22.7

A True

B True

C False

The application may be made by a registered mental nurse or a registered nurse for mental handicap.

D False

The application may be made by the Crown Court.

E False

The application may be made by a police officer.

References/Further Reading

Revision Notes in Psychiatry, pp. 203 and 205.

22.8

For the purposes of the Mental Health Act, an approved doctor is a registered medical practitioner who is approved under Section 12 of the Mental Health Act 1983 by the Secretary of State (with authority being delegated to the Regional Health Authority) as having special experience in the diagnosis or treatment of mental disorder.

A True

The medical recommendation must be by two doctors, at least one of whom is approved under Section 12.

B False

The medical recommendation is by one doctor, who does not need to be approved.

C False

The medical recommendation is by one doctor, who does not need to be approved.

D True

The medical recommendation must be by two doctors, at least one of whom is approved under Section 12.

E True

The medical recommendation must be by two doctors, at least one of whom is approved under Section 12.

References/Further Reading

Revision Notes in Psychiatry, pp. 203, 205 and 206.

22.9

A False

The maximum duration of this Section is 6 months at a time.

B False

The maximum duration of this Section is 6 hours.

C False

The maximum duration of this Section is 72 hours.

D False

The maximum duration of this Section is 28 days at a time.

E False

The maximum duration of this Section is 28 days at a time.

References/Further Reading

Revision Notes in Psychiatry, pp. 203 and 205.

22.10

A True

B False

C True

The nearest relative may discharge the patient, however the hospital managers may prevent this if the doctor in charge of the case certifies that the patient is dangerous, in which case the nearest relative may apply to a Mental Health Review Tribunal (MHRT) within 28 days.

D True

The RMO (Responsible Medical Officer) is the registered medical practitioner in charge of the treatment of the patient, i.e. the consultant psychiatrist; if they are not available, the doctor who is temporarily in charge of the patient's treatment may deputize.

E True

The patient may apply to a MHRT (Mental Health Review Tribunal) within the first 14 days of detention.

References/Further Reading

Bluglass, R. (1983) *A Guide to the Mental Health Act 1983*. Edinburgh: Churchill Livingstone, p. 21.
Revision Notes in Psychiatry, pp. 202 and 203.

23 CLASSIFICATION

Answers

23.1

A True

This is category F30.

B False

F32 is the category depressive episode.

C True

This is category F34.

D False

This is category F29, which is classified under schizophrenia, and schizotypal and delusional disorders.

E True

This is category F31.

References/Further Reading

Revision Notes in Psychiatry, pp. 208–9.

23.2

A False
This is found in DSM-IV as 295.10.

B True
This is F20.0.

C True
This is F20.5.

D True
This is F20.3.

E True
This is F20.6.

References/Further Reading

World Health Organization (1992) *The ICD-10 Classification of Mental and Behavioural Disorders*. Geneva: WHO.

23.3

DSM-IV is the fourth edition of the Diagnostic and Statistical Manual of Mental Disorders, published by the American Psychiatric Association in 1994. Unlike ICD-10, DSM-IV is a multiaxial classification system. A multiaxial evaluation entails the assessment of each patient on several axes, each of which refers to a different class of information.

A False

General medical conditions are classified under axis III.

B False

Mental retardation is classified under axis II.

C False

Psychosocial and environmental problems are classified under axis IV.

D True

E False

These are classified under axis I.

References/Further Reading

Revision Notes in Psychiatry, p. 210.

23.4

A False

Anxious (avoidant) personality disorder occurs as a diagnosis in ICD-10 as F60.6. In DSM-IV, avoidant personality disorder appears.

B True

C False

Anankastic personality disorder occurs as a diagnosis in ICD-10 as F60.5. The corresponding diagnosis in DSM-IV is obsessive–compulsive personality disorder.

D True

E True

References/Further Reading

Revision Notes in Psychiatry, p. 213.

24 PHYSICAL THERAPIES

Answers

This chapter does not consider pharmacotherapy, which is covered in chapters 15–18.

24.1

A True

In 1938 Cerletti and Bini induced seizures electrically.

B True

In 1934 Meduna attempted to treat schizophrenia by inducing seizures chemically.

C False

Kane has carried out important work on, for example, clozapine.

D True

See **A** above.

E False

Charcot carried out important work on, for example, hysteria and hypnosis during the nineteenth century.

References/Further Reading

Revision Notes in Psychiatry, p. 215.

24.2

ECT involves the induction of fits by electrically stimulating the brain briefly. Its main indications are:

* severe depressive illness
* puerperal depressive illness
* mania
* catatonic schizophrenia
* schizoaffective disorder.

   It works rapidly and effectively in the above cases. It is used when pharmacotherapy will not work fast enough, or when the patient is resistant to medication. For example, the life of a severely depressed patient is at risk in the following cases:

* high immediate risk of suicide
* intake of fluid insufficient to maintain renal function
* depressive stupor.

   In such cases the rapid action of ECT would make this an emergency treatment that should be considered seriously. Similarly, the rapid action of ECT may be required in puerperal depressive illnesses in order to reduce the time the mother is unable to look after her baby.

A True

B False

C True

D True

E False

ECT is not a recognized treatment for simple phobias.

References/Further Reading

Revision Notes in Psychiatry, p. 213
Textbook of Psychiatry, pp. 37–8.

24.3

A False

It is the muscle relaxant that is also administered that prevents the body of the patient moving violently during the convulsion; otherwise there would be a risk of the patient sustaining injury, such as a fractured bone.

B False

A bite is placed in the patient's mouth to prevent damage from biting during the convulsion.

C True

The atropine prevents the muscarinic actions of the muscle relaxant.

D False

E True

The atropine reduces secretions.

References/Further Reading

Textbook of Psychiatry, p. 38.
Revision Notes in Psychiatry, pp. 215–16.

24.4

In this form of treatment the patient may be fully deprived of sleep for at least one night or deprived of only rapid eye movement (REM) sleep. A variant involves altering the time at which the patient goes to sleep. The major indication is severe depressive episodes; other indications are given below. It is thought that it leads to a change in the phase relationships of endogenous circadian rhythms; the latter may be out of phase in severe depression.

A True

B True

C True

D False

Phototherapy is a treatment involving exposure to high-intensity light and may be of benefit to patients suffering from seasonal affective disorder (SAD) in whom the onset of depression is in the autumn or winter months.

E True

References/Further Reading

Textbook of Psychiatry, p. 39.
Revision Notes in Psychiatry, p. 216.

24.5

A True

In 1935 Fulton and Jacobsen showed that bilateral ablation of the prefrontal cortex caused chimpanzees to become more placid and less anxious.

B False

C True

See **A** above.

D True

In 1935 (published in 1936), after studying the work of Fulton and Jacobsen, Moniz carried out human frontal leucotomy.

E True

In the nineteenth century, Burckhardt removed post-central, temporal and frontal cortices from patients.

References/Further Reading

Revision Notes in Psychiatry, pp. 216–17.

24.6

Psychosurgery is the selective surgical removal or destruction of central neural tissue in order to influence behaviour. The cerebral tissue removed may be intrinsically normal. At present, it is very rare for psychosurgery to be carried out in Western countries. It is a last-resort treatment, considered only in certain disorders, such as

* chronic severe intractable depression
* chronic severe intractable obsessive–compulsive disorder
* chronic severe intractable anxiety states.

A True

B False

C False

D True

E True

References/Further Reading

Textbook of Psychiatry, p. 39.
Revision Notes in Psychiatry, p. 217.

24.7

Stereotaxic lesions are made in a variety of ways, such as electrocautery, the implantation of radioactive yttrium and thermocoagulation.

A False

B True

This allows radioactive cobalt rays to be directed at the selected target.

C True

D True

E True

References/Further Reading

Revision Notes in Psychiatry, p. 217.
Trimble, M.R. (1996) *Biological Psychiatry*, 2nd edn. Chichester: Wiley, p. 376.

24.8

Some of the specific types of psychosurgical operations that may be used currently include:

- frontal-lobe lesioning
- cingulotomy
- capsulotomy
- subcaudate tractotomy
- limbic tractotomy.

A False

B True

C True

D True

E True

References/Further Reading

Revision Notes in Psychiatry, p. 217.
Trimble, M.R. (1996) *Biological Psychiatry*, 2nd edn. Chichester: Wiley, pp. 376–8.

25 ORGANIC PSYCHIATRY

Answers

25.1

Dementia is characterized by generalized psychological dysfunction of higher cortical functions without impairment of consciousness. In fully developed dementia, the higher cortical functions affected include memory, thinking, orientation, comprehension, calculation, learning capacity, language and judgement. Dementia is an acquired and usually chronic or progressive disorder, although sometimes it may be reversible.

A True

Multiple sclerosis may present with dementia, and this can raise important problems of differential diagnosis. Sometimes the rate of progression of the dementia is very rapid.

B True

When it causes presenile dementia, particularly if physical features are absent, it may prove difficult to differentiate normal-pressure hydrocephalus from Alzheimer's disease.

C True

D False

E False

Intoxication with vitamin D can lead to dementia.

References/Further Reading

Organic Psychiatry, 3rd edn, pp. 693–4.
Revision Notes in Psychiatry, pp. 218–19.
Textbook of Psychiatry, pp. 99–100.

25.2

All true.

Organic mood disorder is a disorder characterized by a change in mood (depressive or (hypo)manic mood), usually accompanied by a change in the overall level of activity, that is caused by organic pathology. There are many causes including psychoactive substance use, medication, endocrinopathies and intracranial causes. Other systemic disorders that may lead to organic mood disorder include:

- pernicious anaemia
- hepatic failure
- renal failure
- rheumatoid arthritis
- systemic lupus erythematosus (SLE)
- neoplasia
- carcinoid syndrome
- viral infections.

References/Further Reading

Revision Notes in Psychiatry, pp. 220–1.

25.3

Organic anxiety disorder is a disorder characterized by the occurrence of the features of generalized anxiety disorder and/or panic disorder that is caused by organic pathology. The symptoms of anxiety include tremor, paraesthesia, choking, palpitations, chest pain, dry mouth, nausea, abdominal pain ('butterflies'), loose motions and increased frequency of micturition. Some of these symptoms, such as paraesthesia, are related to associated hyperventilation. There may be secondary cognitive impairment, for example poor concentration.

A False

B False

C True

D True

E True

References/Further Reading

Revision Notes in Psychiatry, pp. 220–1.
Textbook of Psychiatry, pp. 107 and 108.

25.4

In ICD-10, organic personality disorder is defined as being characterized by a significant alteration of the habitual patterns of behaviour displayed by the subject premorbidly. Such alteration always involves more profoundly the expression of emotions, needs and impulses. Cognition may be defective mostly or exclusively in the areas of planning one's own actions and anticipating their likely personal and social consequences.

The commonest cause is head injury. Other intracranial causes include brain tumours, brain abscesses, subarachnoid haemorrhage, neurosyphilis and epilepsy, particularly when the frontal or temporal lobes are involved. For example, temporal lobe epilepsy may result in aggressive behaviour, hyposexuality or hypersexuality. Other causes of organic personality disorder include Huntington's disease, hepatolenticular degeneration (Wilson's disease), medication such as corticosteroids, psychoactive substance use and endocrinopathies.

A False

B False
This is the active ingredient in evening primrose oil.

C True

D True

E True

References/Further Reading

Revision Notes in Psychiatry, pp. 221–3.

Answers

26.1

Acute intoxication is a transient condition following the administration of a psychoactive substance resulting in disturbances, or in changes in patterns, of physiological, psychological or behavioural functions and responses.

A False

Its intensity is closely related to dose.

B True

C True

D False

Recovery is usually complete.

E False

The effects disappear when the episode has stopped.

References/Further Reading

Revision Notes in Psychiatry, p. 224.

26.2

A True

The dependence syndrome is a cluster of physiological, behavioural and cognitive phenomena in which the use of psychoactive substances takes on a much higher priority for the individual than other behaviours that once had higher value. There is a desire, which is often strong and sometimes overpowering, to take the psychoactive substance(s) on a continuous or periodic basis. Tolerance may or may not be present. Dependence may be psychological, physical or both:

* psychological dependence – a condition in which a psychoactive substance produces a feeling of satisfaction and a psychological drive that requires periodic or continuous administration of the substance in order to produce pleasure or to avoid the psychological discomfort (such as anxiety and depression) of its absence
* physical dependence – an adaptive state that manifests itself by intense physical disturbance when the administration of a psychoactive substance is suspended. There is a desire to take the psychoactive substance in order to avoid the physical symptoms of a withdrawal state occurring (for example, tremor, myalgia and insomnia).

B False

Harmful use is a pattern of psychoactive substance use that is causing damage to health. The damage may be physical (as in cases of hepatitis from the self-administration of injected drugs) or mental (such as episodes of depression secondary to heavy drinking). Harmful use does not refer to adverse social consequences.

C False

Pathological intoxication applies to alcohol.

D True

Confabulation, whereby gaps in memory are unconsciously filled with false memories, is often a feature of the amnesic (or amnestic, dysmnesic, dysmnestic or Korsakov's) syndrome.

E True

In chronic heavy drinkers, a fall in the blood alcohol concentration leads to withdrawal symptoms including delirium tremens (DTs). Hallucinations are often visual and are commonly Lilliputtian in nature. Auditory and tactile hallucinations may also be present.

References/Further Reading

Revision Notes in Psychiatry, pp. 224–6, 230.
Textbook of Psychiatry, pp. 102 and 119.

26.3

F1x.7 Residual and late-onset psychotic disorder is a disorder in which alcohol- or psychoactive substance-induced changes of cognition, affect, personality or behaviour persist beyond the period during which a direct psychoactive substance-related effect might reasonably be assumed to be operating. It is further subdivided into:

- .70 flashbacks
- .71 personality or behaviour disorder
- .72 residual affective disorder
- .73 dementia
- .74 other persisting cognitive impairment
- .75 late-onset psychotic disorder.

A False

B False

C True

Meeting the criteria for organic personality disorder.

D True

Meeting the general criteria for dementia.

E True

May be distinguished from psychotic disorders partly by their episodic nature, frequently of very short duration (seconds or minutes) and by their duplication (sometimes exact) of previous drug-related experiences.

References/Further Reading

Revision Notes in Psychiatry, p. 226

World Health Organization (1992) *The ICD-10 Classification of Mental and Behavioural Disorders.* Geneva: WHO.

26.4

A False

One glass of wine contains approximately 1 unit of alcohol.

B True

C True

D False

One unit of alcohol is approximately 8–10 g of ethanol.

E False

Half-a-pint of standard-strength beer contains approximately 1 unit of alcohol.

References/Further Reading

Revision Notes in Psychiatry, p. 226.

26.5

Excessive alcohol consumption is associated with an increased mortality. Alcohol accounts for one-fifth to one-third of medical admissions to hospital.

A True

Vitamin C deficiency may present with skin haemorrhages and gingivitis.

B True

This refers to cardiac arrhythmias that may occur particularly after binge-drinking.

C True

Alcoholic hepatitis may occur secondary to long-term heavy daily drinking. Liver cell necrosis and inflammation occurs, presenting with right hypochondrial pain and jaundice, sometimes accompanied by ascites and encephalopathy.

D True

Gonadal atrophy affects both men and women.

E True

Alcoholic pseudo-Cushing's syndrome causes obesity, hirsuitism and hypertension.

References/Further Reading

Revision Notes in Psychiatry, pp. 226–9.

26.6

Excessive alcohol consumption during pregnancy can lead to fetal alcohol syndrome.

A True

B False

Microcephaly is a feature of fetal alcohol syndrome.

C False

Low-set ears are a feature of fetal alcohol syndrome.

D True

E True

References/Further Reading

Revision Notes in Psychiatry, p. 228.
Textbook of Psychiatry, pp. 122–3.

26.7

The most important clinical features of Wernicke's encephalopathy are

- ophthalmoplegia
- nystagmus
- ataxia
- clouding of consciousness
- peripheral neuropathy.

In its early stages, Wernicke's encephalopathy may be reversible through abstinence and the administration of high doses of thiamine

A True

B True

Petechial haemorrhages occur in the mammillary bodies and less commonly in the:

- walls of the third ventricule
- periaqueductal grey matter
- floor of the fourth ventricle
- inferior colliculi.

C False

D True

E True

References/Further Reading

Revision Notes in Psychiatry, p. 230.

26.8

Wernicke's encephalopathy is caused by severe deficiency of thiamine (vitamin B_1), which in turn is usually caused by alcohol abuse in Western countries. Other causes of Wernicke's encephalopathy include: lesions of the stomach (e.g. gastric carcinoma), duodenum or jejunum causing malabsorption; hyperemesis; and starvation.

A True

B True

C True

D False

E True

References/Further Reading

Revision Notes in Psychiatry, p. 230.

26.9

A False

The mortality is around 5% and is associated with cardiovascular collapse or infection.

B False

Treatment is supportive with fluid and electrolyte replacement, and high-potency vitamins (especially thiamine to prevent an unrecognized Wernicke's encephalopathy progressing to Korsakov's psychosis). In patients who are very agitated, anxious or frightened, oral or intramuscular haloperidol can be used; if there is hepatic failure, then benzodiazepines can be given. Benzodiazepines can also be given for their hypnotic effect at night.

C False

Good, calming nursing care is essential, preferably in a quiet single room. A low level of lighting should be used at night, sufficient to reassure the patient of his or her orientation in place, but not enough to interfere with much-needed sleep.

D True

Autonomic disturbance in delirium tremens can manifest as

* perspiration
* flushing or pallor
* dilated pupils
* a weak rapid pulse
* mild pyrexia.

E False

The EEG typically shows fast activity in delirium tremens, in marked contrast to the picture seen in most other forms of delirium in which slowing of the dominant EEG rhythms is the characteristic pattern.

References/Further Reading

Organic Psychiatry, 3rd edn, p. 601.
Revision Notes in Psychiatry, p. 230.
Textbook of Psychiatry, pp. 88–9.

26.10

The Misuse of Drugs (Supply to Addicts) Regulations 1997 require that only medical practitioners who hold a special licence issued by the Home Secretary may prescribe, administer or supply diamorphine, dipipanone or cocaine in the treatment of drug addiction; other practitioners must refer any addict who requires these drugs to a treatment centre.

A True

This is diamorphine.

B False

C False

This is a Schedule 1 drug that is not normally used medicinally. Possession and supply are prohibited except in accordance with Home Office authority.

D False

This is a Schedule 1 drug that is not normally used medicinally. Possession and supply are prohibited except in accordance with Home Office authority.

E True

References/Further Reading

British National Formulary, No. 35 (March 1998), p. 9.
Revision Notes in Psychiatry, pp. 236–7.

26.11

Under the Misuse of Drugs Act 1971 the penalties applicable to offences involving the activities related to Controlled Drugs, including their manufacture, supply and possession, are graded broadly according to the harmfulness attributable to a drug when it is misused. For this purpose, the drugs are categorized into three classes. The first two of these are:

(1) Class A drugs

- alfentanil
- cocaine
- dextromoramide
- diamorphine
- dipipanone
- lysergide (LSD)
- methadone
- morphine
- opium
- pethidine
- phencyclidine
- class B drugs when prepared for injection.

(2) Class B drugs

- oral amphetamines
- barbiturates
- cannabis
- cannabis resin
- codeine
- ethylmorphine
- glutethimide
- pentazocine
- phenmetrazine
- pholcodine.

A False

This is a class B drug.

B False

Orally administered amphetamines are class B, but when prepared for injection amphetamines are class A.

C False

These are class B drugs.

D False

This is a class C drug.

E False

References/Further Reading

British National Formulary, No. 35 (March 1998), p. 8.
Revision Notes in Psychiatry, p. 236.

26.12

A False

As mentioned in the answer to Question 26.10, far from doctors introducing the majority of opiate addicts to their drug of addiction, under the Misuse of Drugs (Supply to Addicts) Regulations 1997, only medical practitioners who hold a special licence issued by the Home Secretary may prescribe, administer or supply diamorphine, dipipanone or cocaine in the treatment of drug addiction. The increase in the number of opiate addicts may be related to the wider availability of cheap opiates imported from the Middle East.

B False

The male to female ratio is around 2:1.

C False

D False

E False

Most heroin users are aged between 20 and 30 years.

References/Further Reading

Revision Notes in Psychiatry, pp. 236–7.

26.13

A False

Chronic opioid dependence is associated with small pinpoint pupils.

B False

Chronic opioid dependence in men is associated with erectile dysfunction.

C False

Chronic opioid dependence is associated with constipation.

D True

E True

References/Further Reading

Revision Notes in Psychiatry, p. 237.
Textbook of Psychiatry, pp. 131 and 132.

26.14

LSD, lysergic acid diethylamide, is a very powerful hallucinogen.

A False

The acute effects of LSD are usually not accompanied by clouding of consciousness or demonstrable impairment of intellectual processes; indeed, a heightened state of awareness is maintained, and thought processes characteristically remain clear.

B True

C False

The tendon reflexes are often increased.

D True

Synthaesthesia, in which a stimulus in one sensory modality leads to a hallucination in another, often occurs.

E False

Hallucinations are mainly visual, and tactile paraesthesiae, metallic tastes and strange smells are not uncommon. However, auditory hallucinations are rare.

References/Further Reading

Organic Psychiatry, 3rd edn, pp. 620–1.
Revision Notes in Psychiatry, pp. 244–5.

26.15

The major psychoactive substance found in the cannabinoids is δ-9-tetrahydrocannabinol. This group includes substances derived from the cannabis plant, such as marijuana ('grass') and hashish, and synthetic substances that are similar to tetrahydrocannabinol. The commonest route of administration is by smoking as a cigarette ('joints'), but the oral route may also be used with the substance being mixed with food. Cannabinoids do not cause physical dependence, but can give rise to marked psychological dependence. Cannabinoids are very rarely used clinically, for example in reducing the neurological effects of multiple sclerosis. The psychological effects include:

- euphoria
- anxiety or relaxation
- suspiciousness
- the feeling that time is slowed down
- impairment of judgement (so that it can be dangerous for the user to drive a car)
- heightened sensory awareness
- social withdrawal.

The suspiciousness may occasionally develop into persecutory delusions. Depersonalization, derealization and hallucinations have been reported in cases of very high blood cannabinoid levels.

A True

Tetrahydrocannabinols are responsible for most of the psychological effects of cannabis.

B False

Tetrahydrocannabinols are highly lipophilic.

C False

As tetrahydrocannabinols are highly lipophilic they can be detected in the blood up to 20 hours after a single dose.

D True

Hippocampal changes associated with tetrahydrocannabinols that have been found include:

- decreased neuronal density
- increased glial reactivity.

E True

References/Further Reading

Organic Psychiatry, 3rd edn, pp. 612–13.
Revision Notes in Psychiatry, p. 246.

Answers

27.1

A False

Hughlings-Jackson (1931) considered positive symptoms as 'release phenomena' occurring in healthy tissue; negative symptoms were attributed to neuronal loss. Kurt Schneider (1959) emphasized the importance of delusions and hallucinations in defining his first-rank symptoms.

B True

C False

Kraepelin (1896) grouped together catatonia, hebephrenia and the deteriorating paranoid psychoses under the name 'dementia praecox'. Bleuler (1911) later introduced the term 'schizophrenia', and expanded the concept of dementia praecox to include schizophrenia simplex.

D False

Kraepelin considered dementia praecox to be a disease of the brain. Bleuler was influenced by the writings of Sigmund Freud.

E False

Bleuler considered the symptoms of ambivalence, autism, affective incongruity and disturbance of association of thought to be fundamental in schizophrenia (the 'four As'). Delusions and hallucinations assumed secondary status.

References/Further Reading

Revision Notes in Psychiatry, p.249.

27.2

A False

B True

C True

D False

E False

In defining his first-rank symptoms, Schneider stated that, in the absence of organic brain disease, the presence of the following are highly suggestive of schizophrenia:

- auditory hallucinations, with the repeat of thoughts out aloud (e.g. Gedankenlautwerden, écho de la pensée) or in the third person in the form of a running commentary
- delusions of passivity including
  - thought insertion, withdrawal and broadcast
  - made feelings, impulses and actions
- somatic passivity
- delusional perception.

Second-rank symptoms include perplexity, emotional blunting, and other hallucinations and delusions.

References/Further Reading

Revision Notes in Psychiatry, p. 250.

27.3

A False

Diagnostic guidelines require a minimum of one clear symptom (two if less clear-cut) from the following four groups:

1 thought echo and thought alienation;
2 delusions of passivity, delusional perception;
3 auditory hallucinations in the form of a running commentary or discussing the patient, or hallucinatory voices coming from some part of the body;
4 persistent delusions, culturally inappropriate and impossible.

Alternatively, the presence of symptoms from at least two of the following groups is required:

5 formal thought disorder;
6 catatonic behaviour;
7 negative symptoms;
8 significant and persistent change in overall quality of some aspects of personal behaviour, e.g. aimlessness, idleness.

Thus, there is a weighting towards symptoms of the first rank, which are represented in groups 1 to 4.

B False

C True

All subtypes of schizophrenia, except for simple schizophrenia, require the presence of symptoms for most of the time during a period of 1 month or more.

D False

Affective symptoms may occur in schizophrenia. Schizophrenia is not diagnosed if extensive affective symptoms are present unless they postdate the schizophrenic syndrome. If both schizophrenic and affective symptoms develop together and are evenly balanced the diagnosis of schizoaffective disorder is made.

E False

This applies to the residual or chronic schizophrenia subtype. Simple schizophrenia has an insidious onset of decline in functioning. Negative symptoms develop without preceding positive symptoms. Diagnosis requires changes in behaviour over at least a year, with marked loss of interest, idleness and social withdrawal.

References/Further Reading

Revision Notes in Psychiatry, pp. 251–2.
World Health Organization (1992) *The ICD-10 Classification of Mental and Behavioural Disorders*. Geneva: WHO.

27.4

A True

The age of onset is usually between 15 and 25 years.

B False

Affective changes are prominent. Inappropriate giggling and a fatuous affect are common.

C False

The prognosis is poor. This is possibly related to the earlier age of onset and prominence of negative symptoms.

D False

Delusions and hallucinations tend to be fleeting and fragmentary.

E True

Irresponsible behaviour, disorganized thought, rambling speech and mannerisms are also common.

References/Further Reading

Revision Notes in Psychiatry, p. 252.

27.5

A True

B False

The reality distortion syndrome is characterized by delusions and hallucinations. The disorganization syndrome is characterized by disorders of the form of thought and inappropriate affect.

C True

D True

E False

Hypofrontality in schizophrenia is more often seen in chronic patients and is associated with inactivity and catatonic symptoms.

References/Further Reading

Revision Notes in Psychiatry, p. 253.

27.6

A False

Schizophrenia is most common in social classes IV and V.

B False

The prevalence is higher in urban than in rural areas.

The *social drift theory* (Goldberg and Morrison, 1963) postulates that those with schizophrenia migrate to areas where social demand may be less, such as inner city areas.

The *social causation hypothesis* (Castle *et al*, 1993) suggests that an environmental factor of aetiological importance in schizophrenia is more likely to affect those born in the inner city.

C False

The onset of schizophrenia is earlier in men than in women. Earlier onset of schizophrenia is associated with a poorer prognosis.

D False

The incidence of schizophrenia is between 15 and 30 new cases per 100 000 of the population per year.

E True

References/Further Reading

Revision Notes in Psychiatry, p. 254.

27.7

A False

When both parents are affected, the lifetime risk for the development of schizophrenia in their offspring is about 46%. Thus, more than half of their offspring are not likely to develop the disease.

B False

The risk of developing schizophrenia in the offspring of unaffected monozygotic co-twins is the same as the risk of developing schizophrenia in the offspring of the schizophrenic proband.

C True

D True

E False

Some forms of a single major locus of inheritance could exist, but they would account for a very small proportion of cases. To date, no single genetic locus for the development of schizophrenia has been reliably demonstrated.

References/Further Reading

Revision Notes in Psychiatry, p. 255.

27.8

A True

It is thought that this is caused by increased vulnerability to neurodevelopmental damage, which is commoner in men.

B False

This is in fact evidence in favour of the genetic aetiology of schizophrenia.

C True

It is postulated that the winter excess of births in schizophrenia is caused by a seasonal perinatal hazard such as a viral infection.

D False

E True

These are thought to originate early in the second trimester of pregnancy. It is also at this time during the pregnancy that it is thought that some factor causes disordered brain development in the fetus that predisposes it to develop schizophrenia at a later time.

References/Further Reading

Revision Notes in Psychiatry, p. 256.

27.9

A False

Expressed emotion is not specific to schizophrenia.

B False

It is assessed using the Camberwell Family Interview.

C True

D True

Leff *et al.* (1990) studied levels of expressed emotion in first-contact schizophrenic patients in rural India. At one-year follow up, a dramatic reduction in the expressed emotion in relatives had occurred. It was concluded that the better outcome of this cohort of schizophrenic patients was partly attributable to tolerance and acceptance by family members.

E True

References/Further Reading

Revision Notes in Psychiatry, pp. 257 and 385.

27.10

A False

Only auditory hallucinations of the first rank would support the diagnosis of schizophrenia. These include auditory hallucinations in the third person, in the form of a running commentary and speaking the thoughts out aloud.

B False

Although they may be present they are not diagnostic.

C False

D True

This is a Schneiderian first-rank symptom.

E True

This is a Schneiderian first-rank symptom.

References/Further reading

Revision Notes in Psychiatry, p. 250.

27.11

A False

The ventricle–brain ratio is greater in schizophrenic patients than in controls.

B True

Post-mortem studies have demonstrated reduced brain length in schizophrenic patients compared with controls.

C True

This was demonstrated by Johnstone *et al.* in 1976 when CT scans of the brains of chronically hospitalized patients revealed larger lateral ventricles than those of controls.

D True

E True

References/Further reading

Revision Notes in Psychiatry, p. 259.

27.12

A True

One of the features distinguishing them from conventional neuroleptics.

B False

In the acute situation, the aim is to sedate the patient, thus minimizing the risk of harm to the patient and to others. In this situation, a conventional neuroleptic in moderate dose is used in combination with a fast-acting benzodiazepine. It may be necessary to use the parenteral route for administration if the patient is too disturbed to co-operate with oral administration. Care must be taken in deciding upon the dose of neuroleptic used in this situation. The first-pass effect is significant with neuroleptics, and therefore the parenteral dose is lower than the oral dose for a given effect. Additionally, the choice of benzodiazepine in this situation requires the knowledge that diazepam is poorly and erratically absorbed from the intramuscular route. If diazepam is used, it should be administered intravenously or rectally for rapid and reliable absorption. Lorazepam is commonly used in this situation as it is rapidly absorbed from the intramuscular route and is short acting.

In the heavily sedated patient, the nursing staff should be instructed to maintain close observations, with particular attention to respirations.

C True

D False

Atypical antipsychotics have a reduced potential for extrapyramidal side-effects and tardive dyskinesia, but are not without other side-effects. For example, the atypical drug clozapine has an increased likelihood of inducing agranulocytosis compared with conventional drugs. Convulsions and weight gain are also common.

E True

One of the features distinguishing them from conventional neuroleptics.

References/Further reading

Revision Notes in Psychiatry, p. 260.

27.13

A False

Forty to sixty per cent of schizophrenic patients are non-compliant with prescribed oral medication.

B False

Depot neuroleptics increase compliance and reduce relapse rates.

C False

Occasionally electroconvulsive therapy is used in schizophrenia, particularly in a stuporose or highly excited patient.

D True

E False

Extrapyramidal side-effects occur in up to 90% of patients taking conventional neuroleptic medication.

References/Further reading

Revision Notes in Psychiatry, pp. 260–1.

27.14

A False

B True

This is a feature of an acute brain syndrome and should prompt a search for an underlying physical cause.

C False

This is a Schneiderian first-rank symptom and in the absence of organic brain disease is highly suggestive of schizophrenia.

D True

These are commonly seen in delirium tremens and should prompt a search for other features of this or other acute brain syndromes. Delirium tremens is caused by sudden withdrawal from alcohol in a dependent drinker. It is characterized by disorientation, fluctuating conscious level, intensely fearful affect, hallucinations (often visual, commonly Lilliputian), misperceptions, tremor, restlessness and autonomic overactivity.

Visual hallucinations may occur in affective disorder and schizophrenia, but should always raise the possibility of organic disorder.

E True

This describes a state in which there is a restriction of consciousness with relatively well-ordered behaviour. The commonest cause is epilepsy.

References/Further reading

Revision Notes in Psychiatry, p. 230.
Hamilton, M. (ed.) (1985) *Fish's Clinical Psychopathology,* 2nd edn. Bristol: Wright.

27.15

A False

B False

C False

D True

E False

Florid psychotic symptoms, especially if sudden in onset, do not carry the poor prognosis associated with negative symptoms, particularly of insidious onset.

References/Further reading

Revision Notes in Psychiatry, p. 261.

27.16

A True

B True

The essential feature of this delusional disorder is that a person who is familiar to the patient is believed to have been replaced by a double. Also known as illusion of doubles or l'illusion de sosies.

C False

Cotard's syndrome is also called délire de négation. Erotomania is also called de Clérambault's syndrome.

D False

Othello syndrome is also known as pathological (delusional) jealousy. If the condition is not amenable to treatment (which it often is not), there may be a risk of violence to the object of attention (often this is the patient's partner). It may in some circumstances be best to recommend that the couple separate.

E True

This is a nihilistic delusional disorder. It can be secondary to severe depression or to an organic disorder.

References/Further reading

Revision Notes in Psychiatry, pp. 88 and 262–3.

27.17

A False

The prognosis is poorer for the depressive subtype.

B True

Kasanin introduced the term 'schizoaffective psychosis'. It described a condition of sudden acute onset, good premorbid functioning, with both affective and schizophrenic symptoms.

C False

At least one-third of schizophrenics have depressive symptoms. ICD-10 requires both affective and schizophrenic symptoms to be equally prominent within the same episode of illness.

D True

E False

This would be the conclusion of the binary theorists. Continuum theorists consider psychosis to vary along a continuum, with schizophrenia and manic depression at opposing poles, and schizoaffective disorder somewhere in between.

References/Further reading

Revision Notes in Psychiatry, pp. 263–4.

27.18

A True

This is a rare autosomal recessive condition that sometimes produces a schizophrenia-like psychosis. It is an autosomal recessive disorder of copper metabolism, involving low serum caeruloplasmin, overabsorption of dietary copper, low serum copper and high urinary copper. Copper is deposited in liver, basal ganglia, cerebrum, eyes (Kayser–Fleischer rings), renal tubules and bones. Diagnosis is confirmed by blood caeruloplasmin estimation, and measurement of urinary excretion of copper.

B True

A rare disorder caused by chronic alcohol intake is alcoholic hallucinosis. This is characterized by auditory hallucinations in clear consciousness.

C False

The stimulation of opiate receptors produces analgesia, euphoria, hypotension, bradycardia and respiratory depression.

D True

Particularly temporal lobe epilepsy.

E False

This is a disease characterized by relapsing iritis associated with oral and genital ulceration.

27.19

A False

These changes are commoner in individuals who showed an abnormal personality or social impairment in childhood.

B True

C True

D True

E True

27.20

A False

This applies to all patients who have been detained under Sections 3, 37, 41 and 47.

B True

This requires that: a key worker is allocated; a 'care plan' is drawn up that is based upon a 'needs assessment'; and a review date is established.

C True

About a quarter of first-episode patients will not go on to relapse, and it is therefore worthwhile in this group to reduce antipsychotic medication after a period of 6 months to 1 year. In the case of those who repeatedly relapse, it is recommended that they remain on treatment in the long term, although there is scope for a dose reduction over time.

D True

The advice of the DVLA to doctors is that those patients who have recently recovered from an acute psychotic episode with hospitalization should not drive for 6 months. The licence is likely to be restored if the patient remains symptom free during this period and if they demonstrate that they can comply safely with medication and show insight into their condition. Loss of insight or judgement will lead to a recommendation for the licence to be refused or revoked.

E False

Depot neuroleptics increase compliance and reduce relapse rates.

References/Further reading

Revision Notes in Psychiatry, pp. 196 and 260.

Answers

28.1

A False

Manic episodes are divided into hypomania, mania without psychotic symptoms and mania with psychotic symptoms. Hypomania describes a persistent elevated mood, increased energy and activity, feelings of well-being, reduced need for sleep. It specifies that there are no hallucinations or delusions.

B False

A symptom duration of 2 weeks is required.

C True

Patients who have repeated episodes of mania resemble those who also have depressive episodes in terms of their family history, premorbid personality, age of onset and prognosis.

D False

Manic episodes usually last a median duration of 4 months, while depressive episodes tend to last longer, with a median length of about 6 months, although they may persist for over a year, particularly in the elderly.

E True

This is possible in a mixed affective episode. Both sets of symptoms should be prominent for the greater part of the episode of illness, and the episode should last for at least 2 weeks.

References/Further reading

Revision Notes in Psychiatry, p. 268.
World Health Organization (1992) *Tenth Revision of the International Classification of Diseases.* Geneva: WHO.

28.2

A False

This is more suggestive of a reactive form of depression, whereas early morning awakening is more suggestive of an endogenous form of depression.

B True

C False

This is common to both forms of depression.

D True

E True

The Newcastle school (Roth 1950s) distinguished endogenous from reactive types of depression. The endogenous form was thought to be biological in origin, with psychomotor retardation or agitation, loss of weight, anhedonia, early morning awakening and diurnal mood variation. The reactive form was thought to be of psychological origin, with anxiety, irritability, initial insomnia and persistent reactivity of mood.

Kendall (1965) failed to find a point of rarity in symptomatology between neurotic/psychotic depression and therefore concluded that there were no essential differences between them.

References/Further reading

Revision Notes in Psychiatry, p. 269.

28.3

A False

The sex ratio in bipolar mood disorder is equal. Unipolar depression is more common in women.

B False

Bipolar depression has an more acute onset, which is up to 15 years earlier than unipolar depression on average.

C True

D False

No difference is observed in the sleep EEGs of these two groups.

E True

References/Further reading

Revision Notes in Psychiatry, p. 269.

28.4

A False

This refers to major depression superimposed upon dysthymia.

B False

Although the patient in a depressive stupor is unresponsive, akinetic and mute, they are fully conscious, and after an episode they can recall the events that took place at the time.

C True

D True

Rapid cycling is the term used to describe those bipolar patients who have four or more affective episodes in a year. It is commoner in women and predicts poorer prognosis.

E True

This can occur and may present as 'masked depression' in which somatic symptoms are more likely to be complained of than mood symptoms. It is more common in those unable to articulate their emotions, e.g. those with dementia or learning disability. Diurnal variation in abnormal behaviour may mirror diurnal variation of mood.

References/Further reading

Revision Notes in Psychiatry, p. 269.

28.5

A False

Normal grief has three phases. The stunned phase lasts from a few hours to 2 weeks. This gives way to the mourning phase, which yields after several weeks to the phase of acceptance and adjustment.

B True

These occur particularly during the mourning phase which results in intense yearning and autonomic symptoms.

C False

Grief typically lasts about 6 months.

D True

E True

A typical grief is divided by Parkes (1985) into:

- unexpected grief syndrome
- ambivalent grief syndrome
- chronic grief.

References/Further reading

Revision Notes in Psychiatry, p. 270.

28.6

A False

Brown and Harris found that 15% of urban women had severe depressive symptoms and there was a higher prevalence in working-class than in middle-class women.

B True

C True

The lifetime risk is 5–12% in men and 9–26% in women.

D True

The average age of onset for bipolar disorder is in the mid-twenties, whereas the average age of onset for unipolar depression is in the late thirties.

E False

There is a higher incidence of depression in those who are not married.

References/Further reading

Revision Notes in Psychiatry, p. 270.

28.7

A False

In bipolar probands there is an increased risk of both bipolar and unipolar disorder in first-degree relatives.

B True

C True

A MZ/DZ concordance ratio for bipolar disorder of 79:19 compares with 54:24 for unipolar disorder.

D False

In linkage studies of complex diseases such as affective disorder spurious linkage may be produced because of misclassification and misspecification of the disease model.

E True

In adoptees with bipolar disorder, 28% of biological parents suffer from a mood disorder. In comparison, 26% of the biological parents of non-adoptees suffer from a mood disorder.

References/Further reading

Revision Notes in Psychiatry, p. 271.

28.8

A True

B True

C True

Attention and concentration are commonly impaired in severe depression, which can result in a failure to lay down memory. The result is an apparent disturbance of memory. The patient may fear that they are dementing or losing their mind. Clinical tests of memory are usually normal and impairment of attention and concentration is often detected upon clinical testing.

D True

Reduced sleep is usual in severe depression, particularly with early morning awakening, however sometimes depression can result in reversed neurovegetative symptoms, such as hypersomnia, hyperphagia and weight gain. This is referred to as atypical depression.

E True

References/Further reading

Revision Notes in Psychiatry, p. 270.

28.9

A False

These are compatible with the diagnosis of an affective disorder. They are not symptoms of the first rank.

B False

This is a nihilistic delusion that suggests Cotard's syndrome. It is usually secondary to a very severe depression although it can also be secondary to an organic disorder.

C True

This is a Schneiderian symptom of the first rank, which, in the absence of an organic brain condition, is highly suggestive of schizophrenia.

D True

This suggests passivity of action, which is a Schneiderian symptom of the first rank.

E False

References/Further reading

Revision Notes in Psychiatry, pp. 250 and 263.

28.10

A False

Although high expressed emotion in the families of depressed patients has been shown to increase the risks of relapse as has earlier been shown in schizophrenia, the effect of reducing the number of hours depressed people spend in contact with their relatives does not mitigate this effect, unlike in schizophrenia.

B False

Patients maintained on the full effective dose of antidepressant have proportionately fewer relapses than those whose dose is cut down to a lower maintenance level.

C True

ECT is used in the treatment of resistant mania or manic stupor. It is more commonly used in depression, either for those patients who have proved resistant to drug treatment or for those patients whose depression is life-threatening.

D True

Sudden withdrawal of lithium can result in rebound mania, an effect that can be minimized by a gradual reduction in dose. Premature withdrawal of lithium in bipolar patients results in a 28-fold increase in recurrences over 36 months compared with those patients left on lithium.

E False

Delusional depression is best treated with a combination of antidepressants and antipsychotics.

References/Further reading

Revision Notes in Psychiatry, pp. 275–6.

28.11

A True

B False

Shallowness, lability of affect and inappropriate jocularity (Witzelsucht) are encountered.

C True

D True

Over 80% of patients with Cushing's syndrome develop affective illness during the course of the disorder.

E True

References/Further reading

Revision Notes in Psychiatry, pp. 272 and 411.

28.12

A False

It is more common in men than in women. Parasuicide is commoner in women, especially those aged under 35 years.

B False

Negative associations with suicide include religious devoutness, having lots of children and at times of war.

C True

Risk of suicide increases, more among men than women, during the 5 years after the death of a parent or spouse.

D True

E True

Lability of mood, aggressiveness, impulsivity, alienation from peers, and associated alcohol and substance misuse are high-risk factors.

References/Further reading

Revision Notes in Psychiatry, pp. 278–9.

29.1

A True

After puberty there is an excess in women.

B False

Psychoanalytic psychotherapy has not been shown to be efficacious in the treatment of the neurotic disorders. Pharmacological interventions and cognitive and/or behavioural therapy are generally the treatments of choice.

C True

There is an increased mortality in severe neurotic disorder. The relative risk of death in the decade following treatment for neurosis is 1.7. Suicide is the biggest cause of increased mortality (relative risk 6.1). There is also a major excess of deaths from nervous, circulatory and respiratory disease.

D False

Tyrer randomly assigned various neurotic groups to diazepam, dothiepin, cognitive-behavioural therapy, placebo and a self-help treatment programme. No difference in treatment response between diagnostic groups was found. Diazepam was less effective than dothiepin, cognitive-behavioural therapy, or self-help, which were of similar efficacy in all groups.

E False

Freud suggested that libidinous impulses reaching the ego generate anxiety; repression and symptom formation follow.

References/Further reading

Revision Notes in Psychiatry, pp. 283–4.

29.2

A True

B False

C False

It is out of proportion to objective risk.

D False

It is specific, i.e. anxiety is evoked predominantly by certain well-defined situations. If fear is generalized (free-floating), it is not phobic.

E True

References/Further reading

Revision Notes in Psychiatry, p. 285.

29.3

A False

The sex ratio in social phobia is equal. Other phobic anxiety disorders are more common in women (agarophobia 75%, simple phobia 95%).

B False

Anticipatory anxiety is experienced when the phobic individual contemplates the feared situation or object.

C True

Seligman's preparedness theory states that anxiety is more easily conditioned to certain stimuli such as heights, snakes, spiders, and is resistant to extinction. Prepared stimuli were dangerous to primitive man and may have been acquired by natural selection.

D False

Childhood phobias are always improved after 5 years. In adult phobias, 40% are better and 40% are worse after 5 years.

E False

Using benzodiazepines reduces the level of fear when exposed to the stimulus, thus inhibiting the process of habituation.

References/Further reading

Revision Notes in Psychiatry, pp. 285–6.

29.4

A False

The diagnostic reliability of generalized anxiety disorder is lower than that of other anxiety disorders.

B False

Age of onset is earlier (majority before 20 years) and more gradual than other anxiety disorders.

C True

Torgerson (1983) demonstrated that probands with generalized anxiety disorder had lost their parents by death far more often than probands with panic disorder, suggesting that environmental factors contribute a higher vulnerability for the development of generalized anxiety disorder.

D True

Continuous feelings of nervousness, trembling, muscular tension, sweating, light-headedness, palpitations, dizziness and epigastric discomfort are also common.

E True

References/Further reading

Revision Notes in Psychiatry, p. 290.
Torgerson, S. (1983) Genetic factors in anxiety disorders. *Archives of General Psychiatry* **40**, 1085–9.

29.5

A False

They usually cause distress and interfere with activities. Obsessional thoughts, images and impulses are unpleasantly repetitive.

B False

They are present most days for at least 2 successive weeks causing distress or interfering with activities.

C True

D True

E False

Obsessional symptoms developing in the presence of schizophrenia, Tourette's syndrome or organic mental disorder are regarded as part of these conditions (ICD-10).

References/Further reading

Revision Notes in Psychiatry, p. 291.

29.6

A False

OCD is thought to represent regression to the anal-training stage of development.

B True

Caudate metabolic rate is reduced after treatment with drugs or behaviour therapy in those patients responsive to treatment, with change in symptom ratings correlating significantly with right caudate change.

C False

Antidepressants with selective serotonergic properties show greater efficacy in the treatment of OCD than those without selective serotonergic properties. Clomipramine has serotonergic properties, whereas maprotiline is a specific noradrenaline reuptake inhibitor devoid of serotonergic activity. Thus, patients with OCD are more likely to benefit from treatment with clomipramine.

D True

Antidepressants are effective in the short-term treatment of OCD, but relapse often follows discontinuation of treatment.

E False

The presence of symptoms involving the need for symmetry and exactness indicate a poorer prognosis. Other poorer prognostic factors include male sex, early onset, a family history of OCD, and the presence of hopelessness, hallucinations or delusions.

References/Further reading

Revision Notes in Psychiatry, pp. 291–3.

29.7

A False

Panic disorder involves recurrent unpredictable attacks of severe anxiety lasting usually for only a few minutes.

B False

This is more suggestive of generalized anxiety disorder.

C True

D False

This suggests that agarophobia is the diagnosis. Agarophobia may or may not be associated with panic attacks.

E True

There is a sudden onset, and the following may be experienced: palpitations, chest pain, choking, depersonalization, derealization, together with a secondary fear of dying, losing control or going mad. It often results in a hurried exit and persistent fear of another attack.

References/Further reading

Revision Notes in Psychiatry, p. 287.

29.8

A True

B True

C False

This is usually seen in schizophrenia.

D False

In neurotic illness, insight is usually preserved into the abnormal nature of the experience. This is more likely to be lost in psychotic illness, where behaviour can be observed to be more bizarre and disturbed, and is more likely to contravene social norms.

E False

A stimulus in one sensory modality produces a perception in another sensory modality, e.g. auditory stimulus such as music is experienced as a visual perception such as colours. This is commonly induced by hallucinogenic drugs, typically LSD. It occurs uncommonly in some people who are otherwise well.

29.9

A True

There are similarities between opioid withdrawal and PTSD, leading to speculation that opioid function is disturbed in PTSD. Stress-induced analgesia is reversible by nalaxone infusion in veterans exposed to a traumatic stimulus.

B False

Viewing the dead body of a relative after a disaster is predictive of lower PTSD.

C False

MAOIs and tricyclic antidepressants are particularly helpful for intrusive symptoms, and SSRIs are helpful for avoidant symptoms. Carbamazepine, propranolol and clonidine reduce arousal and intrusive symptoms. Fluoxetine and lithium reduce explosiveness and improve mood. Buspirone may lessen fear-induced startle.

There is an almost total lack of response to placebo in chronic PTSD.

D False

This is true of an acute stress reaction. PTSD usually arises within 6 months as a delayed and/or protracted response to a stressful event of an exceptionally threatening nature.

E True

This is the case even when there was no premorbid tendency to abuse substances.

References/Further reading

Revision Notes in Psychiatry, pp. 293–4.

29.10

A True

Approximate answers. The patient appears to deliberately pass over the correct answer and to select a false answer (which would be easily recognizable as such, even to a child), e.g. What colour is grass? Answer: Blue.

B False

There is subsequent amnesia for the period during which the symptoms were manifest.

C False

Hysterical conversion may occur.

D True

These commonly occur.

E False

This is thought echo and is a first-rank symptom of schizophrenia.

References/Further reading

Revision Notes in Psychiatry, p. 297.

30 DISORDERS SPECIFIC TO WOMEN

Answers

30.1

Psychiatric disorders that are more common in women than in men include:

- senile dementia
- dysthymia
- anxiety and phobic disorders
- dissociative disorders
- anorexia nervosa
- bulimia nervosa
- deliberate self-harm.

A True

B False
This is more common in men.

C True

D True

E False
This is around eight times more common in men than in women.

References/Further Reading

Textbook of Psychiatry, p. 232.

30.2

A True

There is also an increase in suicide during the premenstrual period.

B True

Psychiatric hospital admissions are increased premenstrually, suggesting that premenstrual syndrome may exacerbate pre-existing psychiatric disorder. Mothers are also more likely to take their children to see their general practitioner during the premenstrual period.

C True

There is an increase in both shoplifting and violent crimes during the premenstrual period.

D False

Poor academic performance is more common during the premenstrual period.

E True

References/Further Reading

Textbook of Psychiatry, p. 232.

30.3

A True

Global premenstrual syndrome scores show a much higher concordance rate for monozygotic twins (of 0.55 in the study published by Condon, 1993) compared with dizygotic twins (0.28).

B True

Highly significant correlations between mother and daughter have been reported on a variety of menstrual variables, including premenstrual tension.

C False

Women with type A behaviour experience around 50% more premenstrual syndrome symptoms than women with non-coronary-prone type B behaviour.

D False

Premenstrual symptoms are more common in those around 30 years of age.

E False

The prevalence may increase with increasing parity.

References/Further Reading

Condon, J.T. (1993) The presynaptic-menstrual syndrome: a twin study. *British Journal of Psychiatry* **162**, 481–6.
Revision Notes in Psychiatry, pp. 302–3.

30.4

Miscarriage occurs in 12–15% of clinically recognized pregnancies. Recognized physical causes include:

- fetal chromosomal abnormality
- uterine malformation
- cervical incompetence
- trauma
- infection
- endocrine disorder
- toxins
- irradiation
- immune dysfunction.

A True

O'Hare and Creed (1995) studied the relationship between life events and miscarriage in 48 case–control pairs matched for known predictors of miscarriage. They found that the miscarriage group were more likely to have experienced:

- a severe life event in the 3 months preceding miscarriage
- a major social difficulty
- life events of severe short-term threat in the 2 weeks immediately beforehand.

Fifty-four per cent of the miscarriage group had experienced some psychosocial stress, compared with only 15% of controls.

B True

C False

Miscarriage is associated with having few social contacts.

D True

About a half of all known miscarriages are associated with fetal chromosomal abnormalities.

E True

References/Further Reading

O'Hare, T. and Creed, F. (1995) Life events and miscarriage. *British Journal of Psychiatry* **167**, 799–805.
Revision Notes in Psychiatry, p. 305.

30.5

Postnatal blues constitute a brief psychological disturbance, characterized by tearfulness, emotional lability and confusion in mothers occurring in the first few days after childbirth. There is some evidence of links with biological factors including:

- history of pre-menstrual tension
- serum calcium levels
- monoamines, serum tryptophan, platelet α_2-adrenoceptors
- progesterone withdrawal after delivery.

A False

Postnatal blues peak at the third to fifth day post partum.

B True

C False

It occurs in about 50% of women after childbirth.

D True

Postnatal blues have been positively associated with:

- poor social adjustment
- poor marital relationship
- high scores on EPI neuroticism scale
- fear of labour
- anxious and depressed mood during pregnancy.

E False

A significant association has not been demonstrated between developing postnatal blues and life events.

References/Further Reading

Revision Notes in Psychiatry, p. 307.
Textbook of Psychiatry, p. 240.

30.6

Postnatal depression is a depressive illness not qualitatively different from non-psychotic depression in other settings. It is characterized by low mood, reduced self-esteem, tearfulness, anxiety particularly about the baby's health and an inability to cope. Mothers may experience reduced affection for their baby and may have difficulty breast feeding.

A False

Postnatal depression occurs in 10–15% of post-partum women.

B True

C True

Those women who are emotionally unstable in the first week after childbirth are at an increased risk of developing postnatal depression.

D False

Postnatal depression is not associated with parity.

E False

There is little evidence for genetic factors being of importance in the aetiology of postnatal depression.

References/Further Reading

Revision Notes in Psychiatry, pp. 307–8.
Textbook of Psychiatry, pp. 238–9.

30.7

The following are more frequent in the children of mothers suffering postnatal depression:

- insecure attachment
- behaviour problems
- difficulties in expressive language
- fewer positive, and more negative facial expressions
- mild cognitive abnormalities
- less affective sharing
- less initial sociability.

   Furthermore, social and marital difficulties are often associated with reduced quality of mother–child interaction.

A False

B True

C True

D False

E True

References/Further Reading

Revision Notes in Psychiatry, p. 309.

30.8

The risk of developing a psychotic illness is increased twenty-fold in the first post-partum month. Certain symptoms that are distinctive are:

- abrupt onset, within the first 2 weeks of childbirth
- marked perplexity, but no detectable cognitive impairment
- rapid fluctuations in mental state, sometimes from hour to hour
- marked restlessness, fear and insomnia
- delusions, hallucinations and disturbed behaviour develop rapidly.

A False

Characteristically there is a lucid period followed by a prodromal period of 2–3 days, during which insomnia, irritability and restlessness may occur, with refusal of food. This is then followed by an acute onset of marked perplexity and a rapidly fluctuating clinical picture until the exact nature of the psychosis becomes clear. Onset is usually within the first 2 weeks; the nature and timing are similar to those of post-operative psychosis.

B False

Puerperal psychosis is not a unitary or specific form of psychosis. In order of frequency of their occurrence (highest first), it may be:

- a depressive psychosis
- schizophreniform/schizophrenia
- a manic episode
- an organic psychosis, e.g. delirium.

A few organic psychoses are caused by cerebral thrombosis. About 70% of puerperal psychoses are affective psychoses and around 25% are schizophreniform.

C False

The risk of a subsequent further episode of psychosis is between 1 in 5 and 1 in 3 in any future puerperal periods.

D False

Most mothers require admission to hospital, not only because of the severity and associated behavioural disturbance of their psychosis, but also for the protection of the baby from neglect, mishandling or violence. There is a significant risk of suicide and infanticide.

E False

In breast-feeding mothers, lithium is contraindicated because it is excreted into breast milk and is toxic to the baby.

References/Further Reading

Revision Notes in Psychiatry, pp. 309–11.
Textbook of Psychiatry, pp. 235–7.

31 SEXUAL DISORDERS

Answers

31.1

This question refers to the ICD-10 diagnosis F52.11 Lack of sexual enjoyment.

A True

This complaint is much more common in women than in men.

B False

Orgasm is experienced but there is a lack of appropriate pleasure.

C True

D False

'Failure of genital response' is a separate ICD-10 diagnosis, namely F52.2. In men with failure of genital response, the principal problem is erectile dysfunction, i.e. difficulty in developing or maintaining an erection suitable for satisfactory sexual intercourse. In women with failure of genital response, the principal problem is vaginal dryness or failure of lubrication.

E True

Sexual responses occur normally.

References/Further Reading

Revision Notes in Psychiatry, p. 317.

31.2

Penile erection is a neurovascular phenomenon requiring intact arterial supply and intact venous valves, allowing cavernosal pressures to rise to those approaching systolic blood pressures. Vascular changes are brought about by the parasympathetic autonomic nervous system (S2,3,4) influenced by tactile stimuli and central limbic and cognitive mechanisms. Psychic erections are mediated by thoracic sympathetic outflow, whereas reflex erections result from sacral parasympathetic outflow. Androgens also influence erection, particularly those occurring in sleep, via the limbic system. Studies with community samples indicate that the prevalence of male erectile disorder is around 4–9%.

A True

These cause hyperprolactinaemia.

B True

Diabetes causes a combination of arteriopathy and neuropathy. Two-thirds of diabetic men have erectile impotence. Of these, it is complete in two-thirds and partial in the remaining third. A few also complain of other difficulties, such as premature ejaculation. The onset is insidious, and the course progressive with a marked decline in sexual activity and desire.

C True

In this disease, there is progressive fibrosis in the tunica albuginea and sometimes also in the cavernosa, resulting in curvature of the penis on erection.

D True

This is lead poisoning.

E True

References/Further Reading

Revision Notes in Psychiatry, pp. 318–19.
Puri, B.K. and Weppner, G.J. (1989) *Self-assessment for Psychiatry Examinations.* Edinburgh: Churchill Livingstone, pp. 35 and 99.

31.3

Orgasm, seminal emission and ejaculation are physiologically distinct processes, and are potentially separable. Ejaculation is forceful expulsion of semen from the urethra. If semen is released from the urethra without force it is emission. Before orgasm the male becomes aware that ejaculation is imminent and it follows within 1–3 seconds, 'ejaculatory inevitability'. Ejaculation and emission are mediated by the α-adrenergic sympathetic nervous system. Androgens have a role, as the first sexual consequence of castration is inability to ejaculate, which is rapidly restored with androgen replacement. In severe premature ejaculation, emission alone may occur with no ejaculatory component, minimal or absent orgasm and a long refractory period. In youth, men have a tendency to ejaculate quickly. This usually diminishes with increasing age owing to increasing control with experience, an ability to recognize the approach of ejaculatory inevitability, dampening in responsiveness and lessening of novelty, which arises in a stable relationship.

A True

Anxiety promotes emission but inhibits orgasm, and thus plays a crucial role in premature ejaculation.

B True

Education in ejaculatory control using the pause (stop–start) technique is the treatment of choice. During sensate focus exercises, the male, when he predicts that he will ejaculate shortly, asks his partner to stop, allows his arousal level to subside slightly and then returns to being caressed, repeating the process again when arousal increases.

C True

If difficulty is experienced using the pause (stop–start) technique, then the squeeze technique is used. Just before ejaculation becomes inevitable, stimulation is stopped and the tip of the penis is grasped firmly for about 10 seconds, reducing the reflex ejaculatory response.

D False

The opposite side-effect of delayed orgasm occurs with SSRIs such as fluoxetine. Indeed, such drugs are sometimes used as a treatment in men with premature ejaculation.

E False

Studies with community samples indicate prevalence of 36–38% for premature ejaculation.

References/Further Reading

Revision Notes in Psychiatry, pp. 321–2.

31.4

The final stage of sexual excitement may be orgasm. In both sexes if no orgasm occurs, there is a slow resolution of the physical and psychological changes associated with sexual excitement. Apart from ejaculation, for which there is no female counterpart, the correlates of orgasm are similar in the sexes. Heart rate and blood pressure increase, and there is a sudden increase in skeletal muscle activity involving almost all parts of the body. Rhythmic muscle contractions in the male genital tract expel semen; in women there is transient rhythmical contraction of the uterus and vagina. Psychologically there is an instant sense of relief; at its most extreme there can be virtual loss of consciousness, and relaxation ensues. The exact mechanism of orgasm is not known. In addition to local spinal mechanisms, central nervous activity is also involved. EEG recordings during intense orgasm show changes that have been likened to those occurring during epileptic fits. In orgasmic dysfunction (ICD-10 F52.3) orgasm either does not occur or is markedly delayed.

A False

Orgasmic dysfunction is more common in women than in men.

B True

Opiates appear to have a direct inhibitory effect.

C True

Female anorgasmia has been reported in association with tricyclic, MAOI and SSRI antidepressants, and neuroleptic drugs.

D True

E True

Sociocultural expectations and deficits in skills and sexual techniques are the two most important factors present in most cases. Direct masturbation training is the treatment of choice. Treatment may take place in individual, couple or group settings. Tasks include relaxation, fantasizing and masturbation. The treatment is often successful, but generalization of orgasm induced by masturbation to that induced by intercourse does not always occur.

References/Further Reading

Revision Notes in Psychiatry, pp. 322–3.

31.5

When sexually aroused, the upper two-thirds of the vagina is lax and capacious, while the lower third is closely invested by the surrounding musculature of the pelvic floor. The strongest of these muscles is the levator ani, which forms a U-shaped sling around the posterior and lateral vaginal wall. Intense spasm in a nulliparous woman can virtually occlude the vagina. If these muscles are too tense, vaginal entry is impaired and painful, a condition known as vaginismus. A vicious circle ensues; pain or anticipation of pain causes further muscle contraction thereby increasing the likelihood of experiencing pain.

A False

Vaginismus may be a secondary reaction to some local cause of pain, in which case the ICD-10 category of non-organic vaginismus should not be used.

B False

The squeeze technique is used to treat premature ejaculation in men (see Question 31.3).

C True

It has been found that around 10% of women presenting to a sexual disorders clinic have a primary presentation of vaginismus.

D True

In managing this condition, the emphasis is placed upon helping the woman to gain comfort in exploring her own genitalia and inserting her finger into her vagina. Finger insertion may be all that is required, combined with sensate focus techniques. Additional dilatation may be required using graded dilators. Initially, this is carried out on her own, with the partner being included when her confidence has increased.

E True

References/Further Reading

Revision Notes in Psychiatry, pp. 323–4.

31.6

Dual-role transvestism is the wearing of clothes of the opposite sex for part of the individual's existence in order to enjoy the temporary experience of membership of the opposite sex, but without any desire for a more permanent sex change or associated surgical reassignment. It is categorized in ICD-10 as F64.1.

A False

No sexual excitement accompanies the cross-dressing, which distinguishes dual-role transvestism (ICD-10 F64.1) from fetishistic transvestism (F65.1).

B False

C False

D False

E False

References/Further Reading

Revision Notes in Psychiatry, p. 324.

31.7

Gender identity disorder of childhood (ICD-10 F64.2) refers to disorders, usually first manifest during early childhood (and always well before puberty), characterized by a persistent and intense distress about assigned sex, together with a desire to be (or insistence that one is) of the other sex.

A False

It always first manifests before puberty.

B False

In both sexes, in gender identity disorder of childhood there may be repudiation of the anatomical structures of their own sex, but this is an uncommon, probably rare, manifestation.

C False

The cross-dressing does not cause sexual excitement (unlike fetishistic transvestism in adults).

D True

Boys with this disorder may have a very strong desire to participate in the games and past-times of girls, and female dolls are often their favourite toys.

E True

Between one- and two-thirds of boys with gender identity disorder of childhood show homosexual orientation during and after adolescence. However very few exhibit trans-sexualism in later life, although most adults with trans-sexualism report having had a gender identity problem in childhood. Some girls retain male gender identification in adolescence and some go on to homosexual orientation. Most, however, do not.

References/Further Reading

Revision Notes in Psychiatry, p. 324.
World Health Organization (1992) *The ICD-10 Classification of Mental and Behavioural Disorders.* Geneva: WHO.

31.8

Exhibitionism (ICD-10 F65.2) is a recurrent or persistent tendency to expose the genitalia to strangers (usually of the opposite sex) or to people in public places, without inviting or intending closer contact.

A False

Exhibitionism is almost entirely limited to heterosexual men, exhibiting to adult or adolescent women, usually from a safe distance in a public place.

B True

C True

There is usually sexual excitement at the time of the exposure and the act is commonly followed by masturbation.

D True

Most exhibitionists find their urges difficult to control and ego-alien.

E True

References/Further Reading

Revision Notes in Psychiatry, p. 325.
World Health Organization (1992) *The ICD-10 Classification of Mental and Behavioural Disorders.* Geneva: WHO.

31.9

A False

B True

This refers to rubbing up against people for sexual stimulation in crowded public places.

C False

This is the ICD-10 category F52.10 and is a form of sexual dysfunction in which the prospect of sexual interaction with a partner is associated with strong negative feelings and produces sufficient fear or anxiety that sexual activity is avoided.

D True

This refers to the use of anoxia for intensifying sexual excitement.

E True

This refers to making obsene telephone calls.

References/Further Reading

Revision Notes in Psychiatry, p. 325.

World Health Organization (1992) *The ICD-10 Classification of Mental and Behavioural Disorders*. Geneva: WHO.

31.10

Rape is unlawful sexual intercourse with a woman by force or against her will. Rapists are not a homogeneous group.

A True

Situational stress rapists are otherwise sexually normal. These individuals commit rape when under extreme situational stress. They experience much guilt and remorse afterwards.

B False

C False

D True

Sociopathic rapists have a poor social adjustment with criminality, a poor work record, substance abuse and unstable relationships. Rapes are often impulsive, with immediate gratification with little regard to the consequences. Threats of violence are common.

E True

Sexually inadequate rapists are shy, timid and insecure. They lack social skills. The rapes are often planned, and perpetrated against attractive or sexually threatening woman.
    Other types of rapists that are recognized include:

• *Sadistic rapist*
There is a deep-rooted hatred of women arising from early relationships. The object of the rape is infliction of humiliation and suffering; intercourse may be trivial in comparison to humiliating acts and serious injuries inflicted.The rapes are often carefully planned with precautions being taken to avoid detection.

• *Psychotic rapist*
These are a very small proportion of rapists.The rapes are often bizarre and violent.

References/Further Reading

Revision Notes in Psychiatry, p. 326.

Answers

32.1

Hypersomnia is defined in ICD-10 as a condition of either excessive daytime sleepiness and sleep attacks (not accounted for by an inadequate amount of sleep) or prolonged transition to the fully aroused state upon awakening.

A False

Cataplexy may occur in narcolepsy but not in non-organic hypersomnia.

B False

Sleep paralysis may occur in narcolepsy but not in non-organic hypersomnia.

C False

Hypnagogic hallucinations may occur in narcolepsy but not in non-organic hypersomnia.

D False

Sleep attacks are resistible in non-organic hypersomnia but irresistible in narcolepsy.

E True

References/Further Reading

Revision Notes in Psychiatry, pp. 331–2.
Textbook of Psychiatry, pp. 264–5.
World Health Organization (1992) *The ICD-10 Classification of Mental and Behavioural Disorders*. Geneva: WHO.

32.2

A True

B False

The duration of attacks is typically less than 1 hour each in the case of narcolepsy, but over 1 hour in the case of hypersomnia.

C True

D False

Daytime sleep attacks rarely occur in unusual places in the case of hypersomnia, whereas in narcolepsy they often take place in unusual circumstances.

E True

In daytime sleep attacks caused by hypersomnia, the EEG typically has a non-REM onset, although a sleep-onset REM EEG is more likely to be seen when the patient is suffering from depression or drug withdrawal. The EEG in daytime sleep attacks resulting from narcolepsy typically shows sleep-onset REM.

References/Further Reading

Revision Notes in Psychiatry, pp. 331–2.
Textbook of Psychiatry, pp. 264–5.
World Health Organization (1992) *The ICD-10 Classification of Mental and Behavioural Disorders.* Geneva: WHO.

32.3

The parasomnias are phenomena occurring as part of or alongside sleep. They include:

- sleepwalking
- night terrors
- nightmares
- bruxism
- nocturnal enuresis
- headbanging
- sleep paralysis
- nocturnal painful erections
- cluster headache
- physical symptomatology occurring at night, e.g. paroxysmal nocturnal dyspnoea and sleep epilepsy
- sleep myoclonus.

A False

B False

C True

This is also known as jacatio capitis nocturnus.

D False

E True

This is teeth grinding.

References/Further Reading

Revision Notes in Psychiatry, pp. 332 and 333.
Textbook of Psychiatry, pp. 266–9.

32.4

Sleepwalking or somnambulism (ICD-10 F51.3) is a state of altered consciousness in which phenomena of sleep and wakefulness are combined.

A False

During a sleepwalking episode the individual arises from bed, usually during the first third of nocturnal sleep, and walks about, exhibiting low levels of awareness, reactivity and motor skill.

B False

Most attacks last for less than 10 minutes, although some may last for half an hour or more. Spontaneous awakening sometimes occurs, but usually the subject returns to bed and continues normal sleep.

C False

Dream recall is not reported, and there is usually complete amnesia for what has transpired.

D False

It tends to occur in the deepest stages of sleep (stages 3 and 4), and so may be considered to be a disorder of arousal.

E False

The great majority of cases occur in children.

References/Further Reading

Organic Psychiatry, 3rd edn, pp. 735–7.
Revision Notes in Psychiatry, pp. 332–3.
Textbook of Psychiatry, pp. 266–8.
World Health Organization (1992) *The ICD-10 Classification of Mental and Behavioural Disorders.* Geneva: WHO.

32.5

Sleep terrors (ICD-10 F51.4) or night terrors are nocturnal episodes of extreme terror and panic associated with intense vocalization, motility and high levels of autonomic discharge.

A True

Sleep terrors arise out of stages 3 and 4 of non-REM sleep.

B True

The individual sits up or gets up with a panicky scream, usually during the first third of nocturnal sleep, often rushing to the door as if trying to escape, although he or she very seldom leaves the room.

C True

D False

The episodes typically last 1–10 minutes.

E True

References/Further Reading

Organic Psychiatry, 3rd edn, p. 737.
Revision Notes in Psychiatry, pp. 333–4.
Textbook of Psychiatry, pp. 268–9.
World Health Organization (1992) *The ICD-10 Classification of Mental and Behavioural Disorders.* Geneva: WHO.

32.6

Nightmares (ICD-10 F51.5) are dream experiences loaded with anxiety or fear, of which the individual has very detailed recall. The dream experiences are extremely vivid and usually include themes involving threats to survival, security or self-esteem. Often there is a recurrence of the same or similar frightening nightmare themes.

A False

Nightmares occur during phases of REM sleep.

B False

The awakening may occur at any time during the sleep period, but typically during the second half of sleep.

C True

During a typical episode there is a degree of autonomic discharge.

D False

During a typical episode there is no appreciable body motility.

E False

During a typical episode there is no appreciable vocalization.

References/Further Reading

Revision Notes in Psychiatry, pp. 334–5.
Textbook of Psychiatry, pp. 268–9.
World Health Organization (1992) *The ICD-10 Classification of Mental and Behavioural Disorders.* Geneva: WHO.

32.7

Sleep paralysis consists of attacks of transient inability to move that emerge in the stage between wakefulness and sleep.

A False

The onset is abrupt, with the patient suddenly aware that he or she can neither speak nor move.

B False

Attacks of sleep paralysis typically occur while falling asleep, both at night and with daytime sleep attacks. More rarely they occur during awakening.

C True

The paralysis is flaccid and usually complete, although some patients can open their eyes or even cry out briefly.

D True

The episodes are brief, lasting several seconds and rarely more than one minute.

E True

Hallucinatory voices or sounds sometimes accompany the attack and may cause the patient to fear that he or she is going to be harmed or attacked.

References/Further Reading

Organic Psychiatry, 3rd edn, p. 723.

32.8

This is a rare syndrome of periodic somnolence, often lasting for days or weeks at a time, and associated with intense hunger. Irritability, excitement and motor unrest characterize the somnolent phases.

A False

When awake patients eat voraciously, typically consuming any food in sight. This has been termed megaphagia.

B False

Incontinence does not occur. The patient sleeps excessively by day and night, rousing only to eat or to empty their bladder and bowels.

C False

Hypersexuality may be observed during the waking phases of megaphagia in around a quarter of cases.

D True

E False

References/Further Reading

Organic Psychiatry, 3rd edn, pp. 732–3.

Answers

33.1

The term psychopathy originally included all personality disorders. The term became restricted in the USA to antisocial personality-disordered people and was brought to the UK with that meaning by Henderson in 1939.

A True

These are people who have high ability combined with their severe personality disorder, such as Lawrence of Arabia and the Renaissance sculptor Cellini.

B False

C False

D True

E False

A third kind of psychopathic personality distinguished by Henderson, in addition to aggressive and creative psychopaths, was those who were predominantly inadequate. These included pathological liars, swindlers and conmen.

References/Further Reading

Revision Notes in Psychiatry, p. 336.
Textbook of Psychiatry, pp. 277–8.

33.2

A False

The concept of manie sans délire is associated with Pinel.

B False

The concept of moral insanity is associated with Pritchard

C True

D True

The PAS is the Personality Assessment Schedule.

E False

References/Further Reading

Revision Notes in Psychiatry, p. 336.

33.3

A True

Kelly considered every man to be a scientist, interpreting the world on the basis of past experience. Constructs are created and predictions made accordingly. A system of constructs results, unique in each individual, existing at various levels of consciousness, those formed at earlier developmental stages being unconscious. Each construct has a range of convenience; some are specific, e.g. chewy versus tender, others have a wider range of convenience. Constructs are arranged into hierarchies. Superordinate constructs are central to the individual's sense of identity, subordinate constructs less so. According to the personal construct theory anxiety results when the individual is presented with events outside their range of personal constructs. Hostility comprises imposition of constructs one upon another.

B False

The concept of the repertory grid is associated with Bannister. The repertory grid can be used to assess individual's attitudes with respect to a series of bipolar constructs. (It can also be used to measure formal thought disorder.)

C True

Cattell identified 20 000 words describing personality. Using factor analysis he derived 16 first-order personality factors. Catell's 16 PF test was devised on the basis of this work. Second-order factor analysis resulted in three broad dimensions similar to Eysenck's dimensions:

- sociability
- anxiety
- intelligence.

D False

The Minnesota Multiphasic Personality Inventory (MMPI) is a lengthy inventory in which the subject answers 'true', 'false' or 'cannot say'. It is empirically constructed and measures traits. It is widely used.

E False

The self-theory was devised by Roger. Each individual is said to have a drive to fulfil themselves and develop an ideal self within a phenomenal field of subjective experience. The most important aspect of personality is the congruence between the individual's view of himself and reality and his view of himself compared to the ideal self. If the individual acts at variance to his own self image, anxiety, incongruence and denial result. A congruent individual is able to grow (self-actualization) and achieve their potential both internally and socially.

References/Further Reading

Revision Notes in Psychiatry, pp. 336–9.

33.4

The ICD-10 criteria are:

(a) finds few activities pleasurable;
(b) emotional coldness, detachment or flattened affect;
(c) limited capacity to express feelings;
(d) apparent indifference to praise or criticism;
(e) little interest in sexual experiences with another person;
(f) preference for solitary activities;
(g) preoccupation with fantasy and introspection;
(h) lack of desire for close friends or confiding relationships;
(i) insensitivity to social norms and conventions.

A True

B True

C False

This is a criterion of paranoid personality disorder in ICD-10.

D True

E True

References/Further Reading

Revision Notes in Psychiatry, pp. 339–40.
World Health Organization (1992) *The ICD-10 Classification of Mental and Behavioural Disorders.* Geneva: WHO.

33.5

The ICD-10 criteria are:

(a) self-dramatization, theatricality, exaggerated expression of emotions;
(b) suggestibility, easily influenced by others or by circumstances;
(c) shallow and labile affectivity;
(d) continual seeking for excitement, appreciation by others and activities in which the patient is the centre of attention;
(e) inappropriate seductiveness in appearance or behaviour;
(f) over-concern with physical attractiveness.

A True

B False

This is a criterion of dissocial personality disorder in ICD-10.

C True

D True

E False

This is a criterion of dissocial personality disorder in ICD-10.

References/Further Reading

Revision Notes in Psychiatry, p. 340.

World Health Organization (1992) *The ICD-10 Classification of Mental and Behavioural Disorders.* Geneva: WHO.

33.6

The ICD-10 criteria are:
(a) excessive sensitiveness to setbacks and rebuffs;
(b) tendency to bear grudges persistently;
(c) suspiciousness and a tendency to distort experience by misconstruing the neutral or friendly actions of others as hostile or contemptuous;
(d) a combative and tenacious sense of personal rights out of keeping with the actual situation;
(e) recurrent suspicions, without justification, regarding sexual fidelity of spouse or sexual partner;
(f) tendency to experience excessive self-importance, manifest in a persistent self-referential attitude;
(g) preoccupation with unsubstantiated 'conspiratorial' explanations of events both immediate to the patient and in the world at large.

A False

This is a criterion of schizoid personality disorder in ICD-10.

B False

This is a criterion of dissocial personality disorder in ICD-10.

C True

D False

This is a criterion of histrionic personality disorder in ICD-10.

E True

References/Further Reading

Revision Notes in Psychiatry, pp. 339–40.
World Health Organization (1992) *The ICD-10 Classification of Mental and Behavioural Disorders.* Geneva: WHO.

33.7

The ICD-10 criteria are:

(a) callous unconcern for feelings of others;
(b) gross and persistent irresponsibility and disregard for social norms, rules and obligations;
(c) incapacity to maintain enduring relationships;
(d) low tolerance to frustration; low threshold for aggression and violence;
(e) incapacity to experience guilt or to profit from experience, especially punishment;
(f) marked proneness to blame others.

A False

This is a criterion of paranoid personality disorder in ICD-10.

B False

This is a criterion of paranoid personality disorder in ICD-10.

C True

D True

E True

References/Further Reading

Revision Notes in Psychiatry, pp. 339–40.
World Health Organization (1992) *The ICD-10 Classification of Mental and Behavioural Disorders.* Geneva: WHO.

33.8

The ICD-10 criteria are:

(a) feelings of excessive doubt and caution;
(b) preoccupation with details, rules, lists, order, organization and schedule;
(c) perfectionism interferes with task completion;
(d) conscientiousness, scrupulousness, undue preoccupation with productivity to exclusion of pleasure and relationships;
(e) pedantic;
(f) rigidity and stubbornness;
(g) insist others submit to their way of doing things, reluctant to allow others to do things;
(h) intrusion of unwelcome, insistent thoughts or impulses.

A True

B False

This is a criterion of dissocial personality disorder in ICD-10.

C True

D False

This is a criterion of histrionic personality disorder in ICD-10.

E True

References/Further Reading

Revision Notes in Psychiatry, pp. 340–1.
World Health Organization (1992) *The ICD-10 Classification of Mental and Behavioural Disorders.* Geneva: WHO.

33.9

The ICD-10 criteria are:

(a) persistent, pervasive tension and apprehension;
(b) believe they are socially inept, unappealing or inferior to others;
(c) preoccupation with being criticized or rejected in social situations;
(d) unwillingness to become involved unless certain of being liked;
(e) restrictions in lifestyle because of need for security;
(f) avoidance of activities involving interpersonal contact because of fear of criticism, disapproval or rejection.

A True

B True

C True

D False

This is a criterion of histrionic personality disorder in ICD-10.

E False

This is a criterion of dissocial personality disorder in ICD-10.

References/Further Reading

Revision Notes in Psychiatry, pp. 340–1.

World Health Organization (1992) *The ICD-10 Classification of Mental and Behavioural Disorders*. Geneva: WHO.

33.10

The ICD-10 criteria are:

(a) allow others to make important life decisions;
(b) subordination of own needs to those of others on whom dependent;
(c) unwillingness to make demands on people on whom dependent;
(d) uncomfortable or helpless when alone, fear inability to care for themselves;
(e) fear of being abandoned;
(f) unable to make decisions without excessive advice from others.

A False

This is a criterion of anankastic personality disorder in ICD-10.

B True

C False

This is a criterion of paranoid personality disorder in ICD-10.

D False

This is a criterion of dissocial personality disorder in ICD-10.

E False

This is a criterion of anankastic personality disorder in ICD-10.

References/Further Reading

Revision Notes in Psychiatry, pp. 339–341.
World Health Organization (1992) *The ICD-10 Classification of Mental and Behavioural Disorders.* Geneva: WHO.

33.11

The DSM-IV criteria for antisocial personality disorder are:

A Pervasive disregard for and violation of rights of others occurring since age 15 years. Three (or more) of the following:
   (1) failure to conform to social norms with respect to lawful behaviours;
   (2) deceitfulness; repeated lying, use of aliases, conning others;
   (3) impulsivity, failure to plan ahead;
   (4) irritability and aggressiveness;
   (5) reckless disregard for safety of self or others;
   (6) consistent irresponsibility; repeated failure to sustain work or honour financial obligations;
   (7) lack of remorse.
B At least age 18 years.
C Evidence of conduct disorder before age 15 years.
D Not exclusively during the course of schizophrenia or mania.

A True

It is twice as prevalent in inner cities as in rural areas.

B False

Antisocial behaviours usually start aged 8–10 years. They do not develop after age 18 years. The highest lifetime prevalence of antisocial personality disorder is in the 25- to 44-year-old group, followed by the 18- to 24-year-old group.

C True

Spontaneous remission may occur in middle age. There is a positive correlation between increasing age and remission rate.

D False

Patients are less likely to be married.

E True

There is a highly significant correlation between antisocial personality disorder and drug and alcohol dependence.

References/Further Reading

Revision Notes in Psychiatry, pp. 342–5.

Answers

34.1

The main epidemiological study of behavioural and emotional problems in preschool children is the Waltham Forest Study in the early 1970s of three-year-olds.

A False

B False

The prevalence of moderate to severe behavioural and emotional problems was found to be 7%, while that of mild behavioural and emotional problems was 15%.

C True

D True

E True

References/Further Reading

Revision Notes in Psychiatry, p. 353.
Textbook of Psychiatry, p. 289.

34.2

A False

The overall point prevalence was 6.8%.

B True

C True

D False

The point prevalence was 2.5%.

E False

It was the other way round, with the overall point prevalence of child psychiatric disorder in inner London being twice that in the Isle of Wight.

References/Further Reading

Revision Notes in Psychiatry, p. 353.
Textbook of Psychiatry, pp. 289–90.

34.3

The ICD-10 classification F93 *'Emotional disorders with onset specific to childhood'* includes:

- separation anxiety disorder of childhood
- phobic anxiety of childhood
- social anxiety disorder of childhood
- sibling rivalry disorder.

A False

This is F92.0, part of *'Mixed disorders of conduct and emotion'*.

B True

This is F93.0.

C False

This is F94.0, part of *'Disorders of social functioning with onset specific to childhood and adolescence'*.

D True

This is F93.1.

E True

This is F93.2.

References/Further Reading

Revision Notes in Psychiatry, p. 354.

34.4

The ICD-10 classification F98 *'Other behavioural and emotional disorders with onset usually occurring in childhood and adolescence'* includes:

- non-organic enuresis
- non-organic encopresis
- feeding disorder of infancy and childhood
- pica of infancy and childhood
- stereotyped movement disorders
- stuttering (stammering)
- cluttering.

A False

This is F90.1, part of *'Hyperkinetic disorders'*.

B False

This is F94.2, part of *'Disorders of social functioning with onset specific to childhood and adolescence'*.

C False

This is included in F95.2.

D True

This is F98.3.

E True

This is F98.1.

References/Further Reading

Revision Notes in Psychiatry, p. 354.

34.5

School refusal is refusal to attend or stay at school because of anxiety and in spite of parental or other pressure.

A False

The sex ratio is approximately equal.

B True

There are three main incidence peak ages

- 5 years – separation anxiety
- 11 years – may be precipitated by the change from junior to secondary school
- 14–16 years – this may be a symptom of a psychiatric disorder

C False

D True

Another possible psychiatric disorder that it may be a symptom of in adolescence is a phobia (such as social phobia).

E True

The Kennedy approach entails a return to school being arranged as soon as possible.

References/Further Reading

Revision Notes in Psychiatry, pp. 355–7.

34.6

Truancy is an important differential diagnosis when making a diagnosis of school refusal. Truancy differs from school refusal in that it is:

- ego-syntonic and intended
- often accompanied by other antisocial symptoms
- more likely to be associated with a family history of antisocial behaviour
- more likely to be associated with poor academic school performance
- more likely to be associated with increased family size.

A False

B False

C True

D True

E True

References/Further Reading

Revision Notes in Psychiatry, pp. 355–6.

34.7

A True

It is commoner in males.

B True

C False

The point prevalence is around 1.7% in the UK. The diagnosis is made far more commonly in the USA.

D True

The cardinal features are:

- impaired attention
- overactivity
- impulsivity.

    These should:

- occur in more than one environmental situation
- begin before the age of 6 years
- be of long duration.

E True

The stimulants methylphenidate, pemoline and dexamphetamine may be used.

References/Further Reading

Revision Notes in Psychiatry, pp. 357–8.
Textbook of Psychiatry, pp. 299–300.

34.8

According to ICD-10 elective mutism is characterized by a marked, emotionally determined selectivity in speaking, such that the child demonstrates their language competence in some situations but fails to speak in other (definable) ones.

A False

The sex ratio is equal.

B True

The prevalence is less than 0.8 per 1000 children.

C True

D False

In general, in the long term, the prognosis is good unless other disorders are also present.

E True

References/Further Reading

Revision Notes in Psychiatry, pp. 359–60.

34.9

A True

The male to female ratio is around 2:1.

B False

The lifetime prevalence is around 1.01–1.6%.

C False

The average age of onset is around 7 years.

D True

The prevalence of multiple tics in first-degree relatives is around 14–24%.

E False

About one-third present initially with vocal tics.

References/Further Reading

Revision Notes in Psychiatry, pp. 360–1.
Textbook of Psychiatry, pp. 306–8.

34.10

According to ICD-10 non-organic encopresis is the repeated voluntary passage of faeces, usually of normal or near-normal consistency, in places not appropriate for that purpose in the individual's own sociocultural setting.

A False

B True

It is three to four times more common in boys than in girls.

C True

In the 12-year-olds, the Isle of Wight study found a prevalence of 1.3% in boys and 0.3% in girls.

D True

Non-organic encopresis may be subdivided into:

- continuous encopresis – bowel control has never been achieved
- discontinuous encopresis – there has been a period of normal bowel control in the past.

E False

In general, the prognosis is very good.

References/Further Reading

Revision Notes in Psychiatry, pp. 363–4.
Textbook of Psychiatry, pp. 311–2.

Answers

35.1

Features of the ICD-10 F71 diagnosis moderate mental retardation include:

- IQ range 35–49
- varying profiles of abilities
- language use and development variable (may be absent)
- often associated with epilepsy, neurological and other disability
- delay in achievement of self-care
- simple practical work
- independent living rarely achieved.

A False

The lower boundary of the IQ range is 35 and not 30.

B False

This is a feature of profound mental retardation.

C True

D True

E False

This is a feature of mild mental retardation.

References/Further Reading

Revision Notes in Psychiatry, p. 365.

35.2

The ICD-10 category F80 *'Specific developmental disorders of speech and language'* includes:

- specific speech articulation disorder
- expressive language disorder
- receptive language disorder
- acquired aphasia with epilepsy.

A True

This is F80.1.

B False

This is F81.0.

C False

This is F81.1.

D False

This is F83.

E True

This is F80.3 and is also known as Landau–Kleffner syndrome.

References/Further Reading

Revision Notes in Psychiatry, p. 366.

35.3

The ICD-10 category F84 *'Pervasive developmental disorders'* includes:

- childhood autism
- atypical autism
- Rett's syndrome
- other childhood disintegrative disorder
- overactive disorder associated with mental retardation and stereotyped movements
- Asperger's syndrome.

A False

B False

This is attention deficit–hyperactivity disorder.

C True

This is F84.2.

D False

E True

This is 84.5.

References/Further Reading

Revision Notes in Psychiatry, p. 366.

35.4

Childhood autism is characterized by the following triad:

- poor or absent social interaction
- language and communication disorder
- restricted and repetitive behaviour.

A False

The male to female ratio is 3–4 to 1.

B True

C True

D True

E False

A lack of socioemotional reciprocity is a feature of childhood autism.

References/Further Reading

Revision Notes in Psychiatry, pp. 367–9.
Textbook of Psychiatry, p. 324.

35.5

A False

Bradycephaly is a clinical feature.

B False

Curvature of the fifth finger is a clinical feature.

C False

The IQ is less than 50 in approximately 85% of cases. It is less than 35 in far fewer than 90% of cases.

D True

E True

References/Further Reading

Revision Notes in Psychiatry, pp. 369–70.

35.6

A True

Elongated facies are a clinical feature, including:

- oedema
- tissue thickening
- prognathism.

B True

A large forehead is a clinical feature.

C False

The skin tends to be soft and velvety.

D True

E True

References/Further Reading

Revision Notes in Psychiatry, p. 370.

36 EATING DISORDERS

Answers

36.1

An ICD-10 definite diagnosis of F50.0 anorexia nervosa requires the presence of all the following:

(a) Body weight maintained at 15% below expected; Quetelet's body mass index is < 17.5 kg m^{-2}.

(b) Weight loss self-induced by avoidance of fattening foods and one or more of following: self-induced vomiting; self-induced purging; excessive exercise; use of appetite suppressants and/or diuretics.

(c) Body-image distortion; a *specific psychopathology* comprising a dread of fatness that persists as an intrusive, over-valued idea. A low weight threshold is imposed oneself.

(d) Amenorrhoea in women; loss of sexual interest and potency in men. Endocrine disorder of hypothalamic–pituitary–gonadal axis (HPA), elevated growth hormone and cortisol levels, abnormal peripheral metabolism of thyroid hormone and abnormalities of insulin secretion.

(e) If the onset is prepubertal, the sequence of pubertal events is delayed or arrested. Puberty is often completed with recovery, but menarche is late.

A True

B False

C False

> Quetelet's body mass index = mass(kg)/[height(m)]^2.

D True

E True

References/Further Reading

Revision Notes in Psychiatry, p. 372.

36.2

Physical signs and complications of anorexia nervosa include

- ematiation
- slowed metabolic rate; low blood pressure, slow pulse
- lanugo
- cardiac arrhythmias and failure
- peripheral oedema
- amenorrhoea/loss of libido
- reproductive system atrophy, shrunken uterus and ovaries with cystic multifollicular ovarian changes
- osteoporosis from low calcium intake and absorption, reduced oestrogen and increased cortisol secretion; bone pain and deformity; bone density reduces with increasing years of amenorrhoea, pathological fractures after about 10 years
- hypoglycaemia
- dehydration
- hypothermia, cold intolerance
- seizures
- delayed gastric emptying
- acute gastric dilatation
- pancreatitis
- tetany
- degeneration of myenteric plexus of bowel; cathartic colon; constipation
- reduced growth, delayed puberty
- cardiac and skeletal muscle wasting
- purpura secondary to reduced collagen in skin and bone marrow suppression
- mitral valve prolapse
- proximal myopathy
- impaired liver function
- impaired renal function (due to chronic dehydration and hypokalemia)
- diffuse EEG abnormalities reflecting metabolic encephalopathy, may result from fluid and electrolyte disturbances
- brain imaging: increase in the ventricular–brain ratio secondary to starvation.

A True

B True

C True

D False

Hypotension rather than hypertension tends to be seen in anorexia nervosa.

E False

Constipation is a feature of anorexia nervosa.

References/Further Reading

Revision Notes in Psychiatry, p. 373.

36.3

Blood biochemical abnormalities that commonly occur in anorexia nervosa include:

- hypokalaemia (cardiac arrhythmias, cardiac arrest, renal damage)
- hypoglycaemia
- metabolic alkalosis
- hypomagnesaemia
- hypozincaemia
- hypophosphataemia
- raised serum amylase
- hypercholesterolaemia
- hypercarotaemia.

A False

B True

C False

D False

E True

References/Further Reading

Revision Notes in Psychiatry, p. 374.

36.4

Haematological abnormalities commonly seen in anorexia nervosa include:

- leucopenia with relative lymphocytosis
- normochromic normocytic anaemia.

A False

B False

C True

D True

E True

References/Further Reading

Revision Notes in Psychiatry, p. 374.

36.5

A True

B True

C False

The prevalence rate is probably around ten times lower than this.

D False

There is a higher prevalence in higher socioeconomic classes and a significant association with greater parental education.

E True

References/Further Reading

Revision Notes in Psychiatry, p. 374.

36.6

Physical signs commonly occurring in bulimia nervosa that may result from vomiting include:

- dental erosion
- parotid gland enlargement
- Russell's sign
- oedema
- conjunctival haemorrhages
- oesophageal tears
- ipecacuanha intoxication causing cardiomyapathy and cardiac failure, usually fatal.

A True

This consists of callouses on the dorsum of the hands following the use of the fingers to induce vomiting.

B True

C True

D True

These result from raised intrathoracic pressure.

E True

This is associated with dental erosion.

References/Further Reading

Revision Notes in Psychiatry, p. 379.

36.7

A True

B False

The average age of onset of bulimia nervosa is 18 years, which is slightly older than that for anorexia nervosa.

C True

The prevalence among adolescent and young adult women is approximately 1–3%.

D True

The lifetime prevalence for strictly defined bulimia nervosa is 1.1% in women and 0.1% in men.

E False

The monozygotic to dizygotic twin concordance rate for narrowly defined bulimia nervosa is 23–9.

References/Further Reading

Revision Notes in Psychiatry, p. 379.

Answers

37.1

The International Pilot Study of Schizophrenia was devised to determine whether schizophrenia could be recognized as the same condition in a wide variety of cultural settings. The Present State Examination was translated into seven languages, and psychiatrists trained in its use interviewed 1200 patients. Diagnoses were then generated using the computer program CATEGO.

A False

It was conducted by the World Health Organization.

B False

The main results were published in 1973.

C True

There were nine centres:

- Columbia
- Czechoslovakia
- Denmark
- India
- Nigeria
- Russia
- Taiwan
- UK
- USA.

D False

E True

The main findings of the study were:

- when the narrow criteria of Schneider's first-rank symptoms were applied, an incidence of schizophrenia was found that did not differ significantly across cultural settings. Therefore schizophrenia is recognizable as the same condition across a wide variety of cultures
- broadly defined schizophrenia has an incidence that differs significantly from one country to another
- the outcome of schizophrenia was found to vary inversely with the social development of the society. Those from developing countries had a better prognosis than those from the developed world.

References/Further Reading

Revision Notes in Psychiatry, p. 384.

37.2

Amok consists of a period of withdrawal, followed by a sudden outburst of homicidal aggression, in which the sufferer will attack anyone within reach. The attack typically lasts several hours until the sufferer is overwhelmed or killed. If alive, he typically passes into a deep sleep or stupor for several days, followed by amnesia for the event.

A True

It was first described in Malays in the mid-sixteenth century. It was believed to have originated in the cultural training for warfare among Malay warriors. Later it became a personal act by an isolated individual, apparently motiveless, but the motive could be understood as restoration of self-esteem or 'face'. Amok was very common in Malaya at the beginning of the nineteenth century, but the incidence reduced when the British took over the administration of Malaya. Today it has virtually disappeared.

It is commonest in Malays, but reports of amok from other countries do exist.

B False

It almost always occurs in men.

C True

D True

E True

Among Malay cases in psychiatric hospitals, the commonest diagnosis is schizophrenia. Depression, acute brain syndrome and hysterical dissociation have also been found in some cases. The majority do not have a mental illness. Attacks are often preceded by interpersonal discord, insults or personal loss, and social drinking.

References/Further Reading

Revision Notes in Psychiatry, pp. 386–7.

37.3

Koro is common in South-East Asia and China and it may occur in epidemic form. It occurs in men and involves the belief of genital retraction with disappearance into the abdomen, accompanied by intense anxiety and fear of impending death. Cases of a similar condition have been described in non-Chinese subjects. In these cases the syndrome is often only partial, such as the belief of genital shrinkage, not necessarily with retraction into the abdomen; usually occurring in the context of another psychiatric disorder and resolving once the underlying illness has been treated. Debate as to the cultural specificity of this disorder continues with some arguing the culturally determined syndrome to be clearly different to the symptom of genital retraction occurring in some non-Chinese psychotic subjects. The development of koro has been associated with psychosexual conflicts, personality factors and cultural beliefs in the context of psychological stress.

A True

B False
It only occurs in men.

C True

D False

E False

References/Further Reading

Revision Notes in Psychiatry, p. 387.
Textbook of Psychiatry, p. 347.

37.4

Dhat is commonly recognized in Indian culture, and is also widespread in Nepal, Sri Lanka, Bangladesh and Pakistan. Vague somatic symptoms occur (fatigue, weakness, anxiety, loss of appetite, guilt, etc.) and sometimes sexual dysfunction (impotence or premature ejaculation), which the subject attributes to the passing of semen in urine as a consequence of excessive indulgence in masturbation or intercourse. Subjects are typically from a rural area, from a family with conservative attitudes towards sex and of average or low socioeconomic status.

A False

B False
This is a disorder of men.

C False

D False

E False
Literacy and religion are unimportant.

References/Further Reading

Revision Notes in Psychiatry, p. 387.

37.5

Windigo is described in North American Indians, and is ascribed to depression, schizophrenia, hysteria or anxiety. It is a disorder in which the subject believes that they have undergone a transformation and become a monster who practises cannibalism. It has been suggested, however, that windigo is in fact a local myth rather than an actual pattern of behaviour.

A False

B True

C True

D False

E False

References/Further Reading

Revision Notes in Psychiatry, p. 387.

37.6

Latah usually begins after a sudden frightening experience in Malay women. It may also occur in North Africa. It is characterized by a response to minimal stimuli that includes:

- exaggerated startles
- coprolalia
- echolalia
- echopraxia
- automatic obedience.

It has been suggested that this is merely one form of what is known to psychologists as the 'hyperstartle reaction' and is universally found.

A True

B True

C True

D True

E True

References/Further Reading

Revision Notes in Psychiatry, pp. 387–8.

37.7

Five symptom types have been described as comprising brain fag syndrome:

- head symptoms – aching, burning, crawling sensations
- eye symptoms – blurring, watering, aching
- difficulty grasping the meaning of spoken or written words
- poor retentivity
- sleepiness on studying.

A False

Brain fag syndrome is a widespread low-grade stress syndrome described in many parts of Africa and also in New Guinea.

B False

It is commonly encountered among students, probably because of the high priority accorded to education in African society; it is particularly prevalent at times that examinations take place.

C True

D True

E False

References/Further Reading

Revision Notes in Psychiatry, p. 388.

Answers

38.1

Changes with ageing that may affect pharmacokinetics include:

- ↓ total body mass
- ↓ proportion of body mass that is composed of water
- ↓ proportion of body mass that is composed of muscle
- ↑ proportion of body mass that is composed of adipose tissue
- ↑ gastric pH
- ↓ rate of gastric emptying
- ↓ blood flow in splanchnic circulation
- ↓ gastrointestinal absorptive surface
- changes in plasma protein concentration – this may be the result of illness
- ↓ metabolically active tissue
- ↓ hepatic biotransformation
- ↓ glomerular filtration rate
- ↓ renal tubular function.

A False

B True

C False

D True

E True

References/Further Reading

Revision Notes in Psychiatry, p. 398.

38.2

With respect to tricyclic antidepressants, with ageing there occurs:

- ↑ plasma half-life
- ↑ steady-state levels
- ↑ volume of distribution
- ↑ postural hypotension

A True

B True

C False

D False

E False

The elderly are particularly prone to antimuscarinic (anticholinergic) side-effects, which may result in acute brain syndromes, urinary retention and glaucoma.

References/Further Reading

Revision Notes in Psychiatry, pp. 398–9.

38.3

Changes in psychological functions, such as mood, personality, behaviour and cognition, are often the first signs of psychiatric illness in the elderly. Various scales have been devised to provide for accurate and objective assessment of all aspects of psychological functioning in the elderly. The simpler tests can be used by non-psychologist disciplines in their assessment and monitoring of the elderly who are mentally ill. Psychologists can help other disciplines in their roles, and take on the psychometric assessments of those patients with confusing or particularly demanding clinical pictures. Psychometric testing quantifies the level and range of ability. Serial measures can be used to monitor the effects of interventions, or to measure the progress of the patient's condition over time. It is essential when any particular test is used in the elderly that it has been validated in the elderly population, and that its predictions have also been validated.

A True

The Kew Cognitive Map can be used to assess parietal lobe function and language functions in patients with dementia.

B False

This is a modified version of the WAIS for use in children between the ages of 5 and 15 years.

C True

The Clifton Assessment Procedures for the Elderly (CAPE) can be used to predict survival, placement, level of disability, and decline in elderly subjects.

D True

The Kendrick Battery was developed to distinguish normal, functionally impaired and demented elderly groups.

E False

This is a modified version of the WAIS for use in children between the ages of 4 and 6 years and 6 months.

References/Further Reading

Revision Notes in Psychiatry, pp. 23, 24, 404–5.

38.4

All true.

Clinical features that occur in the early stage include:

- impaired concentration
- memory impairment
- fatigue and anxiety
- fleeting depression of mood
- exaggeration of pre-existing personality traits
- unusual incidents cause increasing concern
- occasional difficulty with word finding
- altered handwriting
- perseveration of words and phrases

   Clinical features that occur in the intermediate stage include:

- further deterioration in the above
- neurological abnormalities start to appear
- 5–10% develop epilepsy
- apraxias and agnosias develop
- disorientation in time and space
- get lost in familiar surroundings
- speech problems with nominal dysphasia, receptive dysphasia, expressive dysphasia, dysarthria, reduced vocabulary
- groping for words, mispronunciation, reiteration of parts of words (logoclonia), echolalia
- reduced ability to read and write
- concurrent progressive memory loss involving recent and past events
- misidentification (e.g. mirror sign)
- emotional lability
- catastrophic reaction (extreme anxiety and tearfulness when unable to complete a task)
- motor restlessness or inertia.

References/Further Reading

Revision Notes in Psychiatry, p. 407.

38.5

The term leukoaraiosis was used by Hachinski to describe the CT scan appearances of reduced density of white matter. It differs from infarcts in that it affects only white matter, is patchy and diffuse, and is not associated with enlargement of cerebral sulci or ventricles. It is found in non-demented subjects as well as those with degenerative and vascular dementia.

A False

It is a neuroradiological diagnosis.

B False

It is more common in multi-infarct dementia.

C True

D False

E False

It occurs in the white matter.

References/Further Reading

Organic Psychiatry, 3rd edn, pp. 459–60.
Revision Notes in Psychiatry, p. 410.

38.6

The clinical features of Creutzfeldt–Jakob disease include:

* there may be a brief prodromal period of anxiety, depression or hallucinations
* sudden onset and rapid progression of dementia, pyramidal and extrapyramidal deficits presenting usually in the 50- to 60-year-old age group
* physical features include limb spasticity, muscular wasting and fasciculation, tremor, rigidity, choreiathetoid movements, myoclonus, dysarthria and dysphagia
* convulsions may occur.

   In addition to the above classic form, three variant forms are described:

* heidenhain form
* ataxic form
* cortical form.

A False

B True

In the heidenhain form prominent visual defects occur that may result in:

* cortical blindness
* extrapyramidal symptoms
* myoclonus.

C False

D True

In the ataxic form rapidly progressive cerebellar ataxia occurs, with involuntary movements and myoclonic jerks. Finally, muteness and generalized rigidity may result.

E True

In the cortical form, parietal lobe symptoms occur.

References/Further Reading

Revision Notes in Psychiatry, p. 413.

38.7

General paralysis of the insane is a terminal consequence of syphilis. There is marked cerebral atrophy with meningeal thickening resulting from neuronal loss and astrocyte proliferation. The presence of iron pigment in microglia and the perivascular spaces is specific for the disease. Spirochaetes are found in the cortex in 50% of cases.

A False

It usually develops 5–25 years after primary infection with *Treponema pallidum*.

B True

C False

Grandiose delusions are present in only about 10% of cases.

D True

E True

Physically, there is slurred speech, tremor of lips and tongue, and Argyll Robertson pupil in 50% of cases. As the condition progresses, there is increasing leg weakness leading to spastic paralysis.

References/Further Reading

Revision Notes in Psychiatry, p. 415.

Answers

39.1

A False

Juvenile delinquency is law-breaking behaviour by 10- to 20-year-olds.

B False

C True

Factors associated with the development of juvenile delinquency include:

- unsatisfactory child-rearing
- low IQ
- conduct disorder in childhood
- parental criminality
- large family size.

D False

It is associated with a large family size.

E True

References/Further Reading

Revision Notes in Psychiatry, p. 429.
Textbook of Psychiatry, pp. 361–2.

39.2

A False

In the UK, the peak age of offending is 14 years in girls and 17–18 years in boys.

B True

The sex ratio of convicted men to women is approximately 5:1.

C True

D False

There is a peak of offending around the time of the menopause.

E True

References/Further Reading

Revision Notes in Psychiatry, p. 429.
Textbook of Psychiatry, pp. 359–60.

39.3

A False

In England and Wales criminal responsibility starts at the age of 10 years. In Scotland, criminal responsibility starts at the age of 8 years.

B False

It starts at the age of 10 years.

C False

Criminal responsibility is partial (Dolci Incapax) between the ages of 10 and 14 years.

D True

E False

After the age of 14 years an individual is legally responsible for their actions unless caused by

- a mistake
- an accident
- duress
- necessity
- responsibility being affected by mental disorder.

References/Further Reading

Revision Notes in Psychiatry, p. 430.
Textbook of Psychiatry, p. 362.

39.4

All true.

In England and Wales, the outcomes of sentencing of mentally abnormal offenders include:

- the law takes its course, e.g. fine, prison
- conditional discharge or absolute discharge
- a probation order with or without a condition of psychiatric treatment
- detention under the Mental Health Act.

References/Further Reading

Revision Notes in Psychiatry, p. 432.
Textbook of Psychiatry, p. 364.

39.5

A mentally disordered offender is unfit to plead if, at the time of the trial (but not necessarily at the time of the offence), they are unable to carry out one or more of the following:

- instruct counsel
- appreciate the significance of pleading
- challenge a juror
- examine a witness
- understand and follow the evidence of court procedure.

A False

B True

C False

D True

E True

References/Further Reading

Revision Notes in Psychiatry, p. 432.

39.6

Homicide is the killing of another person. In England and Wales, it may be:

- lawful and justifiable
- lawful and excusable
- unlawful
- causing death by dangerous driving.

Unlawful homicide is 'the unlawful killing of any reasonable creature in being and under the Queen's peace, the death following within a year and a day'.

A False

This is a lawful and excusable type of homicide.

B True

Under the Infanticide Acts 1922 and 1938, infanticide refers to the situation in which a woman by any wilful act caused the death of her child under the age of 12 months, but at the time of the act or omission the balance of her mind was disturbed by reason of her not being fully recovered from the effect of giving birth to the child, or the effect of lactation consequent upon the birth of the child.

C True

Murder by persons of malice aforethought, either expressed or implied. This implies full *mens rea* and intent and results in a mandatory life sentence in England and Wales.

D False

This type of homicide is regarded as being lawful and justifiable.

E True

This refers to the situation in which the homicide follows an unlawful act that was threatening harm or was negligent, and was voluntary, i.e. there was no malice aforethought. A manslaughter verdict allows discretionary sentencing and follows from a successful defence of:

- diminished responsibility
- provocation
- part of a suicide pact
- an unlawful act or omission that directly caused the death but that was carried out without intention to cause death or grievous bodily harm.

References/Further Reading

Revision Notes in Psychiatry, p. 433.
Textbook of Psychiatry, pp. 371–3.

39.7

Kleptomania, or pathological stealing, refers to the recurrent failure to resist irresistible impulses to steal objects not needed for personal use nor for their monetary value. The objects may be discarded, given away or hoarded. There is typically an increasing sense of tension before and a sense of gratification during and immediately after the act.

A False

It is classified under ICD-10 F63 *'Habit and impulse disorders'. 'Other disorders of adult personality and behaviour'* is the ICD-10 category F68.

B False

The disorder is generally said to be rare, with fewer than 5% of arrested shoplifters giving a history consistent with kleptomania.

C False

The average age of onset is around 20 years.

D False

The diagnosis is usually made 1 or 2 decades after the average age of onset.

E False

Stealing is carried out without long-term planning and without the assistance of others.

References/Further Reading

Textbook of Psychiatry, pp. 380–1.

39.8

Being a contract, a marriage is void if an individual had a mental disorder at the time of marriage such that the nature of the contract was not appreciated at that time.

A True

B True

The marriage may be annulled if one partner did not disclose that they suffered from epilepsy or a communicable veneral disease before the marriage.

C False

D True

Non-consummation may be used as a reason to annul a marriage.

E True

See **B** above.

Other reasons for which a marriage in England and Wales may be annulled are:

- either party was under the age of 16 years at the time of marriage
- pregnancy by another man at the time of marriage was not disclosed
- one of the partners was forced to agree to the marriage by duress.

References/Further Reading

Revision Notes in Psychiatry, p. 434.